Palliative Neurology

Palliative care affirms the value of holistic support for persons facing death from advanced disease. Its concern embraces the physical, emotional and spiritual components of distress and suffering, and extends to family members, who experience great anxiety and often are forced to undertake a considerable burden of care. Increasingly the approach of palliative care is seen as relevant not only to terminal cancer but also to many other conditions that cannot be cured or lead to death. This handbook provides succinct and practical advice on the management of the major neurological disorders in both their supportive and terminal phases, recognizing that these conditions are increasing in prevalence in virtually every society along with a growing proportion of elderly persons. It demonstrates how the discomforts met with in dementia, stroke, Parkinson's disease, amyotrophic lateral sclerosis (ALS), Huntington's disease, muscular dystrophies and multiple sclerosis benefit also from a comprehensive approach to palliation by interdisciplinary teams.

Palliative

can do for the dying
You don't even have to
hat you are thinking about
burden. As neurologists ... we
r patients just by seeing and talk-

ist P.G. McManis in the final weeks of
esophageal cancer.
el Harper. *Neurology* 2005; 64: 598–9.

ness

palliation includes the attempt to understand the
s and relationships and activities that have, in the
e one who now faces the loss of much that has consti-
self-image and well-being. To help an individual hold
s such as dignity, determination, courage, confidence and
n the face of uncertainty and unpredictability, recurrent
r progressive deterioration is a core clinical responsibility; to
ze and encourage a patient's capacity for humour and love may
more well-being than any number of interventions focused on
cific symptoms.

Ian Maddocks

Contents

Foreword

A scan through recent literature in the two fields of palliative medicine and neurology suggests little overlap in their clinical practice. In the three major palliative care journals published, respectively, in UK, Canada and USA, the primary focus is advanced cancer. Fewer than 5% of papers deal with non-cancer conditions, and most often these are respiratory, cardiac and renal diseases, with only ALS representing neurology care. Similarly, published texts and articles in neurology concern themselves primarily with diagnosis, investigation and active treatment of disease, and include relatively little about end-of-life care and effective symptom management in advanced disease.

A small number of exceptions exist. The publication in 2004 of the text 'Palliative Care and Neurology', a multiple author work coordinated by neurologist Raymond Volz, reflected a new awareness among neurologists that their responsibility in clinical care ought to extend beyond the major hospital, and ensure effective support and symptom management in home and chronic care settings. A little earlier, in 2001, an issue of Neurology Clinics was devoted entirely to palliative care. Although selective in the number of conditions it addressed, it represented a new direction in the field.

There are readily discernible trends in modern neurology practice that will make it difficult for specialist neurologists to be active in promoting and engaging in the delivery of palliation support for persons affected by chronic neurological conditions. The number of those affected persons, especially among the aged, increases steadily, while the number of specialist neurologists is relatively small, and they are busy in office and hospital practice. The provision of palliation support is often necessarily prolonged and burdensome, and falls more on the larger number of general physicians, gerontologists, family physicians and the various paramedical professions. Increasingly, moreover, neurology divides into subspecialities, and in their more narrow areas of interest its practitioners are excited by new potentials for diagnosis and management, occasioned by innovative radiological and stem cell technologies and novel medications. All this makes training in palliative care (and even in general medicine and general neurology?), an option fewer trainee neurologists will see as necessary.

This text contends that the approach and skills of palliative care are relevant and readily transferable to incurable non-cancer conditions, whether for their terminal stages or during the period before the terminal phase is reached. Given the importance of such conditions in neurology, therefore, it behoves the specialist neurologist to accept a responsibility to know something of the new discipline of palliative care, and to be aware of what its approach and operation – palliation – can contribute to the quality of life of neurology patients. Neurologists should also understand how to engage and, if necessary, supervise the deployment of palliation team expertise for the benefit of both individual patients and attending family members.

The potential readership for this text includes all members of such teams – all the professional categories that contribute to care for such persons.

Neurodegenerative conditions are not generally well understood by the lay public, yet families necessarily undertake a major responsibility for care, often over a prolonged period. Family carers of patients may also find this text useful, whether for negotiating care options with professional staff or for advocacy with community resources or employers.

The emphasis is on the maintenance of comfort and function in the face of physical and mental deterioration; the neurological conditions are arranged with relatively brief introductions, giving emphasis to the management of major symptoms. The attitude to be encouraged is one of helping persons live their lives as normally as possible rather than becoming the subjects of 'treatment'.

The plan to write this small text arose from contact with colleagues at Mie University Hospital, Tsu City, in Japan. In that Prefecture, there is a higher incidence of amyotrophic lateral sclerosis (also called motor neurone disease) than in most other parts of the world. Neurologists there, especially Dr Yugo Narita, Dr Norikazu Kawada and their chief, Prof. Shigeki Kuzuhara, encouraged me write to about palliation in neurology, with a view to having the text translated to Japanese. I am grateful to them for this encouragement and support.

As principal author, I must accept responsibility for any errors or deficiencies. Coming to this theme as a palliative care physician based in Adelaide, Australia, I am ignorant concerning specialist neurology. The faults you find here are mine. But I acknowledge with gratitude the advice and the contribution of my consultant fellow–authors who represent a spectrum of neurological practice: Prof. Bruce Brew, Chairman of Neurology at St Vincent's Hospital, Sydney; Dr Heather Waddy, neurologist in private consulting practice in Adelaide and Dr Ian Williams, a consultant neurologist with a particular interest in people affected by chronic neurological conditions and their support in community settings in the UK. Diana Maddocks provided consistent support, critical review and meticulous proof reading.

Ian Maddocks
Adelaide, Australia
May 2005

Note on drugs and abbreviations

The drugs listed throughout the text, and their formulations, are mainly those currently available in Australia, with a few additions drawn from English texts. Due to the variation in drug company names, generic names are used. The doses suggested are for adults.

There are many medications available for the management of symptoms in neurological practice, and frequently several will be suggested as alternatives for treating a particular discomfort. An important part of the practice of palliation is the recognition of individual patient variation, and of the fact that rarely will one medication be satisfactory for assisting comfort in all the patients who have a common symptom.

Each physician will have favourite choices, but each should also be prepared to change and to experiment with possible alternatives.

Symptoms are often multiple, and the list of medications for any patient may be long. While every clinician wishes to avoid unnecessary prescribing and to avoid polypharmacy, it is inevitable that many individuals in the advanced and terminal stages of a neurological illness will be receiving, at the one time, medications for pain, nausea, constipation, anxiety and depression, muscle dysfunction and sleeplessness. Swallowing is often impaired, and formulations that are available for parenteral use, and particularly for S/C injection in the home via an indwelling cannula, assume a special importance.

Where a drug is listed, its various formulations are appended with reference to the dose and type of each.

Using morphine as an example:

- *morphine 1, 2, 5 and 10 mg/ml susp.* indicates that liquid preparations of morphine are available as 1 mg/ml, 2 mg/ml, 5 mg/ml and 10 mg/ml;
- *morphine 5, 10 and 15 mg tab.* 10–20 mg 4 hourly prn indicates the several strengths of immediate release morphine that are available, and the dose range 10–20 mg is suggested for a particular use;

• *morphine 5, 10, 15 and 30 mg/ml inj. (sulphate); 120 mg/1.5 ml (tartrate).*
20–500 mg by S/C infusion per 24 h. Indicates various ampoules
available for parenteral use, and the range of doses that may be
necessary when using a 24 h S/C infusion.

CR or SR: controlled- or sustained-release formulation; bd: twice daily;
tds: three times a day; qid: four times a day; prn: as required; cap.: capsule;
inj.: injection; supp.: suppository; S/C: subcutaneous route; I-V: intravenous
route.

SECTION I

Palliative Management

Introduction to palliation

PALLIATION, PALLIATIVE CARE AND PALLIATIVE MANAGEMENT

These related terms can be distinguished individually.

To use an analgesic for relief of pain, to inject insulin to control diabetes, to inject botulinum toxin for relief of torticollis is to *palliate*, to provide temporary relief.

To invoke *palliative care* is to call upon a newly recognized specialist practice that has evolved primarily for the care of persons with incurable cancer. It is a practice that embodies a philosophy of compassionate concern, one that recruits human and technical resources to provide a cooperating and comprehensive oversight and continuing support to relieve the totality of discomforts (physical, emotional and even spiritual).

Palliative management or the *practice of palliation* takes up the basic philosophy of palliative care, but brings it into fields other than cancer, encouraging the implementation of constructive palliation by any clinical speciality. Palliative management has been neglected in the modern emphasis on triumphs of cure or major disease modification, but it becomes the most appropriate approach to care when it is apparent that a patient's disease cannot be cured, or that the course of that disease cannot be modified in any significant way. The emphasis of professional attention is then on comfort and the maintenance of best possible function.

Palliative management will offer a comprehensive support that addresses the many components of discomfort (physical, emotional and spiritual) that may accompany advanced disease, and will make that support part of the responsibility of care. It will incorporate much of the approach to care that has developed within the speciality of palliative care, and sometimes it may work closely with staff from that speciality, but more often it will not. It will seek to allow the patient maximal opportunity to participate in decisions about what care is required, and where it is best delivered. It will recognize that no one professional can deliver the wide range of interventions that have potential to assist patient and family, and encourage the participation of a multi-disciplinary team equipped to assist care at any site, whether in acute hospital or aged care facility, in the home or in a specialist in-patient unit.

The origin of 'palliation' and 'palliative' is the Latin: *pallium* means a cloak. The term palliation began, it would seem, with the idea of covering over or keeping out a discomfort to make it bearable, as a cloak will hide a disfigurement or will prevent cold air chilling the body. It describes an action that seeks not to reverse the cause of a discomfort, but to shield against its effect; not to bring about a complete restoration or cure, but to provide a shelter within which to find a greater measure of coping and comfort and well-being.

'HOSPICE' AND PALLIATION IN ADVANCED CANCER

The word 'hospice' is commonly used in connection with palliative care, sometimes to indicate a building: '*St Christopher's Hospice*'; sometimes a group of workers: '*the hospice team*'; sometimes a programme: '*The Northern Hospice Service*'.

'Hospice' also has a Latin origin: *hospes*, meaning a guest, or a host who receives a guest. A 'hospice' was an important part of a typical European Monastery one thousand years ago, providing accommodation for travellers, but was also a place where the monks could offer care for sick or indigent persons.

The term 'hospice' was adopted in the modern era by pioneers such as Mary Aikenhead in Dublin, and Cicely Saunders in London for the institutions they established for the care of dying persons, and it became a common name for such places. It remains a favourite word for indicating a building where dying persons receive care, but for other uses it is now commonly replaced by 'palliative care' or 'supportive care'. In many places there are restrictions on the diseases regarded as suitable for referral to a hospice programme or admission to a hospice; for example, a diagnosis of advanced cancer and a prognosis of less than a defined duration (e.g. 6 months).

Palliative care continues to evolve, however, and is increasingly accepting responsibility for conditions other than cancer.

PALLIATIVE MANAGEMENT IN NEUROLOGY: AN INCREASINGLY RECOGNIZED NEED

In the practice of neurology, many degenerative conditions are not accessible to cure and cause major discomforts and much family distress. Many have the additional feature of a prolonged course that entails a heavy continuing burden on the family support and health services involved in care. In Japan, the term for these conditions translates appropriately as '*obstinate diseases*'. The speciality of neurology is a particularly appropriate setting for palliative management.

In the prolonged course of many 'obstinate diseases' it may be possible to distinguish two phases, namely a supportive phase and a terminal phase. The separation of these phases will often be indistinct, however, and palliative interventions may have value in either:

(i) In the '*supportive phase*' management will aim for maintenance of function at the best level, and the relief of discomfort will be directed to that end. This will involve palliative interventions that mitigate the effects of underlying pathology, and provide a temporary relief, allowing the affected person the best opportunity of continuing life as normally as possible. This phase is usually the responsibility of the neurologist and the family physician. For some particular interventions they may call upon the expertise of other specialties: surgery, speech therapy, psychiatry, etc.

(ii) The *terminal phase* starts when it is clear that function is becoming severely impaired, and irreversible further changes are now being recognized which herald the approach of death. This is a time when more demanding personal care is likely to be required, when symptoms may be more difficult to control, when care by family members will need additional support, and the patient may require temporary or long-term admission to an in-patient setting. At this stage, if funding provisions allow and resources are available, palliative management may be enhanced by access to the skills, experience and resources of a multi-disciplinary palliative care service. Often, however, the neurology team or the family doctor and community agencies must accept the major responsibility for the delivery of care.

DIFFERENT TRAJECTORIES OF CARE FOR CANCER AND NEUROLOGICAL DISEASE

Cancer

A common diagram to indicate the timing of the relationship between oncology and palliative care in the management of cancer shows that the diagnosis of cancer and its initial treatments are within the province of the oncologist, who provides a continuing oversight as measures against the cancer (surgery, chemotherapy, radiotherapy and hormonal treatments) are undertaken (Figure 1.1.1).

The early weeks and months following a diagnosis of cancer are often times of optimism and hope, with (usually) some response to treatment. Prognosis, though still uncertain, seems open-ended. Some time later, however, if recurrence of the cancer becomes apparent, and chemotherapy is less effective, patients will be encouraged to accept the multi-disciplinary assistance of a palliative care team.

A palliative care team, by its name and reputation, represents the reality of approaching death, and referral to palliative care often is not easy for individuals and families to accept. Many will recognize, however, the palliative care team promises the patient a skilled and attentive support throughout the final phase of the illness. That support will be multi-dimensional, embracing symptom control, equipment provision, and concern for the emotional and spiritual well-being of the family as well as the patient. It will be offered on a continuing basis at whatever site of care the patient chooses as most appropriate, and will continue as bereavement support for the family, after death has occurred.

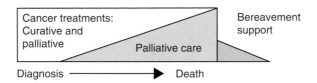

Figure 1.1.1 Relationship of oncology and palliative care.

Neurological diseases

'Obstinate' neurological conditions commonly have a much longer clinical course than is usual with advanced cancer, even though the eventual outcome may also be death. The themes of management in the early 'supportive' stage are those of encouragement, rehabilitation and preservation of function, as well as palliation of symptoms. Supervision is commonly by a neurologist, working within a team structure that includes other health care disciplines. In Figure 1.1.2, the trajectory of a typical degenerative condition is compared with that for advanced cancer and severe respiratory and cardiac diseases. A palliation approach becomes the appropriate response rather late in the course of many cancers, and is less consistently brought into the conduct of care for respiratory and cardiac diseases. For those, the final months and years may be marked by successive crises of acute deterioration, necessitating a series of acute hospital admission for active curative treatments with (hopefully) subsequent recovery after each, but a steady underlying decrease in function, until finally it becomes accepted that further intensive treatment is unlikely to be successful and may be very uncomfortable. Some incurable neurological conditions may follow a terminal pathway similar to cancer or to cardiac disease, with patients not feeling 'ill' until the condition is far advanced; but for other 'obstinate' neurological conditions such as dementia, amyotrophic lateral sclerosis (ALS) or multiple sclerosis (MS), from almost the time of diagnosis, palliation is a close partner with whatever treatments are undertaken to seek to modify the course of the illness.

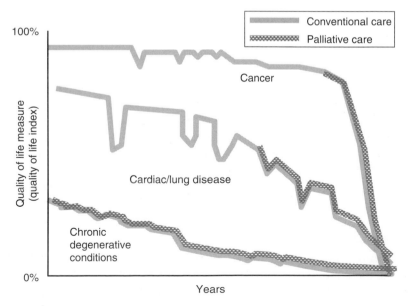

Figure 1.1.2 The pathway of conventional treatments and palliation in major terminal diseases.

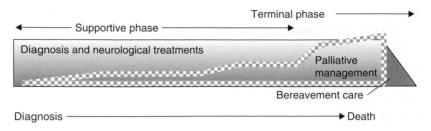

Figure 1.1.3   The relationship of supportive and palliation management phases.

Figure 1.1.3 returns to a comparison with Figure 1.1.1. The boundaries enclosing neurology and palliative management are drawn as less distinct than for oncology and palliative care. Expertise in palliative management will be useful early in the course of the illness, and becomes more and more necessary as the end approaches, when physical abilities are failing, cognition is more impaired, and comfort in all its dimensions becomes more difficult to maintain. The phases labelled 'supportive' and 'terminal' therefore overlap.

By accepting their major role in palliative management, neurologists stand to find new interest and confidence in the management of patients with chronic degenerative conditions. It may lead to a closer partnership with local palliative care teams, offering mutual advantage to both disciplines, and the opportunity for improved care for the many neurology patients who suffer from advanced and terminal disease.

PALLIATION AND NEUROSCIENCE

Around 100 years ago, major advances were made in the understanding of neurological function, as it became possible to assign specific functions to designated areas of the nervous system. Particular nerve tracts and particular collections of neurones in the brain were identified, and anatomy and function could begin to be correlated. This led to understandings of the progression of a stimulus such as pain from the periphery of the body (as with a bruised finger) ascending along nerve trunks, passing through synapses at various points but directed always centrally towards the thalamus and cerebrum where the experience of pain was appreciated, and localized to the site of the stimulus.

It was always clear that this was an inadequate over-simplification. New technologies such as positron emission tomography (PET) scan and functional magnetic resonance imaging (functional MRI) have now made it possible to visualize the simultaneous close interaction of the many elements of the nervous system. We can now recognize a far greater complexity of response to a pain stimulus, with multiple neuronal signals transmitting not only centrally along the recognized ascending tracts, but following descending pathways also, and reverberating within the brain and spinal cord:

> 'A complex barrage of multi-sensory afferent signaling arrives at the brain constantly, and this array varies from moment to moment.
> The signals from [the new stimulus] are relatively minor features of the stream of neural signals that reaches the brain, yet they affect consciousness, causing pain'.
>
> *Chapman CR, Nakamura Y. Pain and consciousness.*
> *Pain Forum 1999; 8:113–23.*

An old way of telling a lay person about the brain was to liken it to a telephone exchange, in which each part of the body had its messages directed to an appropriate part of the cerebrum, where it could be appreciated consciously, and from which responses could be directed and sent out.

A better model for brain function may be something quite chaotic in form (something more akin to a nest of ants in frantic motion), with messages running between all parts in all directions, yet somehow directed and arranged and organized to make sense: sense composed of various orders of complexity and sophistication, and sense that varies from time to time:

> 'Non-conscious and massively distributed central processes integrate the signals from nociceptors with other sensory and affective activity in the brain and various memories and associations'.
>
> *Ibid.*

The patterns that form, moment by moment, in this swirling mass of activity are replaced immediately by others, but there is also potential to store meaningful patterns of activity in some way, making them available for recall or unconscious operation. They will recall past experiences and influences and also frame expectations for both the present and the future.

This modelling of the central nervous system has led to new concepts of consciousness, seeing it as a quality that the brain is constantly revising, elaborating new drafts of awareness, and constructing dynamic representations of reality. In our awareness, nothing is 'actual' or 'true'; it is a construct in which input from the five senses is much influenced by both memory and expectation.

None of this bold reformulation of neurophysiology should be a surprise to practitioners of palliation. They know that the same apparent intensity of stimulus will result in quite different responses in different individuals or in the one person at different times. The 'holistic' approach to palliation that its representatives advocate is one that seeks to maintain, for a suffering individual, an interest in the total context of discomfort, the past experiences, the family connections, the anxieties and fears that affect him, the meanings he is able to give to the current experience. Clinicians try to tune into elements of that person's neural complexity, to appreciate and influence the patterns that are recurring within that nervous system and are causing discomfort. This is no simple task, and it is presumptuous to expect success in bringing comfort. But that is the task, to be undertaken in humility, and as conscientiously as possible.

Compassionate palliative management seeks a close and intimate awareness of a suffering individual's situation. In exploring the potential elements that contribute to that suffering, those who profess palliative management bring their own neural complexities into apposition with those of the patient (utilizing both rigorous clinical assessment and intuition), hoping to *feel* the content of that individual's discomfort, and at the same time measure it in some scientifically acceptable way. It will be good if the caring physician, drawing on available scientific evidence, is, at the same time, aware of the influence of his or her own personality, history and current situation, personal memories and patterns of neural activity, since these clearly affect the perception of the patient's problems.

Sometimes there is little for the physician to offer apart from presence and personality:

> 'One thing I have learned is that the best thing that anyone can do for the dying (or bereaved) individual is to show that you care. ... You don't even have to mention the problem at hand, just show the person that you are thinking about them and therefore are helping to shoulder their burden. As neurologists ... we are obviously providing a lot of comfort for our patients just by seeing and talking to them, even in hopeless cases.'

> *Spoken by distinguished neurologist Philip Geoffrey McManis in the final weeks of his life, prior to his death from oesphageal cancer. Quoted in McManis' obituary by C. Michel Harper. Neurology 2005; 64:598–9.*

External stimuli from many sources also have the potential to be recruited and incorporated in a neural pattern arising from some trauma or pathology, and they can strongly influence the degree to which there is pain or other distress. Fear and anxiety, past distress, an uncomfortable isolated environment or loneliness are all human experiences that can augment suffering, and probably have their effect through modifying neural patterns. Similarly, stimuli of a potentially pleasant nature, such as familiar and meaningful music, touch, massage or attractive odours, the various components of complementary therapy, may become incorporated into complex neural networks and alter them in ways that reduce discomfort. There is already evidence that the neural patterns evoked by pleasing music differ from those evoked by music that is not welcomed. Complementary therapies have the potential to modify neural patterns such as are evoked by pain.

Amazing scientific advances have ensued from active pursuit of analytical methods, but now we have to encourage them to fit into a broader approach to diagnosis and therapy. Palliation, in particular, while it draws enthusiastically on evidence-based medicine, must accept rigorously won evidence as only one component of many that contribute to clinical understanding of the whole of the suffering experienced by an individual.

Palliation in an age of new, more successful therapies

Promising results are being reported for the use of embryonic and adult stem cells for neuro-transplantation in animal models of diseases such as Parkinson's disease. The view that neuronal tissue is immutable is being modified, replacement of nerve cells occurs in specific areas such as the dentate nucleus and the sub-ventricular zone of the lateral ventricles. Response to brain injury by an increase in nerve cell production and regenerative repair has only recently been recognized. Stem cells can invade the cord when introduced into the cerebrospinal fluid (CSF) in rats. Reports from China of symptom improvement in patients with ALS, MS and Parkinson's disease following introduction into the brain of olfactory ensheathing glial (OEG) cells from foetal olfactory bulb tissue are also encouraging.

Many issues remain to be elucidated, but there is a new excitement in neurology as it views the prospect of many new techniques with potential to reverse some hitherto incurable pathologies of the nervous system. That prospect in no way diminishes the need to offer effective palliation.

This small book will have achieved a major aim if it encourages a closer collaboration between scientific neurology, with its confident exploration of new developments in effective treatment, and palliative management, with its comprehensive attention to discomfort. A bi-partisan effort in care offers a brighter horizon of hope for patients afflicted by chronic degenerative disorders of the nervous system.

2

Characteristics of palliation

The following underlying characteristics have been claimed for palliative care. How well do they apply in palliation for an incurable neurological condition?

IT IS PATIENT-CENTRED

Relief of discomfort is the central focus of palliation. An understanding of the underlying pathology remains important for determining the basis of discomforts, and for recognizing where measures aimed at that pathology can improve quality of life, but treatment directed at the underlying disease often is of less importance. Now the assessment and management of the many effects of the disease that diminish the well-being and the dignity of the patient assume prime importance. They include physical discomforts such as weakness and incoordination; emotional frustration from imposed dependency; anxiety about being a burden to others, and spiritual distress with feelings of guilt or unresolved anger, a sense of life losing its meaning, being left without hope for the future. Key elements in human well-being and dignity are the maintenance of a sense of control, and the opportunity to exercise choice. Both are commonly eroded in advanced neurological disease. The term 'existential pain' is sometimes used as a metaphor to indicate suffering that seems to have little connection to physical distress or pain. It is a vague term, thought variously to indicate guilt, isolation through illness, or disappointment and impending separation.

As function deteriorates, friends run out of conversation and commitment dwindles. Although cultural contexts vary, it is not uncommon for persons with chronic neurological diseases to become emotionally and physically isolated as their condition progresses. Many live alone at home, sometimes in very poor conditions, with brief visits from 'carers'. Personal hygiene, laundry and household cleanliness can suffer. In these circumstances people have little control over decisions and become passive. Without effective advocates they are not likely to receive support and may end their lives alone in an inhospitable home or on an acute ward, admitted because of an avoidable complication of a condition recognized too late. At best they may spend their last days in a nursing home cared for by people with little understanding either of the underlying condition or of palliative care.

Those affected by chronic neurological conditions are often physically very dependent and suffer impaired cognition and speech, being restricted in their ability to frame personal wishes or to verbalize them. They may be disruptive and noisy, even violent, and difficult to calm, or conversely may seem dull and uncomplaining. In either case, staff may be tempted to make decisions concerning care without consulting the patient, or may be led to isolate them at the fringes of a medical setting, away from the main ward, perhaps in a side room. There they receive only cursory attention, while patients with interesting diseases or personalities, or those with readily remediable major discomforts, attract more staff interest and time.

It is in meeting the daily basic needs of patients (turning, mobilizing, feeding, washing and toileting) that the fullest appreciation of needs may be achieved. In home settings, family members learn to understand those needs very well; in institutions, staff who accept roles as individual care managers, seeing the same set of patients regularly, can achieve a similar appreciation.

Care in such settings may rely on relatively poorly trained professionals or family members, but they can be the ones best placed to review patient needs and to see that they are anticipated and satisfactorily met. They can achieve also a good understanding of a patient's emotional and intellectual status (and potential), and so be able to introduce creative interventions that not only maintain comfort but also facilitate pleasure and companionship, and offer at least some opportunity for individual choice. It will be wise to recruit such individuals as key participants in the care team, encouraging in them a responsibility to report very clearly their appreciations of patient needs. Reports of their observations may signal a need for more sophisticated assessment and intervention by a physician, for example, to relieve pain, to counteract spasticity, to overcome persistent nausea, to relieve constipation and to support ventilation.

IT PROVIDES TRUTHFUL INFORMATION CONCERNING DISEASE STATUS AND PROGNOSIS

Greater public access to medical information via popular texts and the Internet has raised patient awareness of illness and fuelled greater questioning of medical activity. Societal expectations increasingly advocate the right to know. An increased emphasis on personal autonomy is a relatively recent phenomenon, one that has led to a greater questioning of medical authority throughout all Western societies. Commonly, in Asian traditions (particularly among the older generations) such questioning is less, because to question a superior (or a doctor) is an unacceptable defiance of authority. There, family authority and protection of the patient from bad news has been the rule, but change towards more open exchange is occurring, sometimes spearheaded by informed palliative care practice.

A palliation approach seeks to reduce the distance between staff and patient that hierarchy imposes, and foster a more intimate relationship through careful attention to discomfort. That relationship encourages, and even requires, open and honest exchange at the bedside, and evolves naturally towards greater openness and truth-telling.

The advice concerning truth in political life, offered two centuries ago by the English statesman, Edmund Burke, is relevant to disclosure of medical information:

> 'Falsehood and delusion are allowed in no case whatsoever, but, as in the exercise of all virtues, there is an economy of the truth. It is a sort of temperance, by which a man speaks truth with measure, that he may speak it longer'.
>
> *First of Letters to a fellow MP, 1796. Edmund Burke.*

Clinical assessments that suggest future disappointment or discomfort are not to be withheld or falsified, but offered with care and with sensitivity, if necessarily, a little at a time (see Telling the bad news of ALS in Chapter 5 of Section III p. 156).

IT OFFERS SUPPORT FOR FAMILY MEMBERS

Psychological support

Alongside most individuals with incurable disease there are family members who are experiencing an anticipatory grief, and an anxiety about whether they have the necessary strength and skills to assist in care. It is a time when old family tensions, new disagreements and financial concerns may surface. Decisions concerning sites of care, specific aspects of symptom management, or what, who and how to tell others about the situation may prove difficult to resolve. If a family conference can be arranged with a health team member, it will allow ventilation of concerns and help reach agreement on appropriate decisions.

An important part of the clinical responsibility is ensuring that adequate emotional support is available for carers, whether these are staff in care institutions or family members undertaking home care. The sometimes tedious round of tasks which must be undertaken for patients who can give no thanks needs recognition, as does the low status assigned to continuing care of the aged and disabled within the worlds of medicine and the media. Those family members who undertake care at home need to know that when they are troubled and need advice or assistance they can reach a 'real person', someone who is familiar with their situation and knowledgeable about how to help. A reliable 24-h helpline that can offer advice by telephone in unforeseen crisis events is a significant practical and emotional aid.

Clinicians need to be willing to enter into end-of-life discussions with patients and/or with families as situations suggest, and opportunities allow. Situations that provide triggers for such discussions include:

- open questions by patient or family about what is ahead,
- obvious social or spiritual distress,
- pain or other symptoms difficult to control,
- dysphagia requiring feeding tube support,
- dyspnoea limiting all but minimal activity, or
- a further loss of function in more than one part of the body.

Some end-of-life discussions will inevitably focus on whether to persist with active supportive measures and at what stage it will be advisable and possible to withdraw life-sustaining care (such as tube feeding or assisted ventilation).

Physical support

The care of any person with advanced disease, but particularly frail individuals in whom mobility is much impaired, requires skill and physical strength for the everyday care of hygiene, turning and transferring the dependent patient. Family carers will benefit from education and demonstration of home care techniques, the supply of appropriate equipment and from regular visits by community nurses, allied health staff, social workers, etc. They also need to be thoroughly aware of what is available to assist their work in the local extended care network and have confidence in their ability to recruit assistance when it is needed (see Practical Aspects of Home Care in Chapter 1 of Section V, p. 225).

IT MAINTAINS COMPREHENSIVE CARE

The range of possible symptoms associated with advanced and incurable illness is very wide, and every effort should be made to appreciate, in each individual, the full range of physical, emotional and spiritual discomforts being experienced.

When cure is impossible, symptomatic relief employing non-medical interventions may be at least as important as informed prescribing. The type of mattress or chair, the consistency and taste of food, a choice of music available, the opportunity to move into the sunshine on a fine day, the companionship of loved persons; any of these may facilitate a new level of comfort.

An interest in, and concern for social and spiritual aspects of care – including the effect of a prolonged illness on close relationships, on family finances, on spiritual beliefs and religious attachments – is appropriate. Religion and spirituality are not identical, though they may coexist. A wide range of expressions of spiritual need must be expected in an increasingly multicultural world, and though good understanding across cultural divides may prove difficult to achieve, it begins with a preparedness to listen attentively.

IT ENSURES CONTINUITY OF CARE

A neurological illness, being of longer duration, may involve many changes in function and comfort, and need repeated re-assessment and continuing oversight. Over time, patients may move from one site of care to another, with new clinicians assuming responsibility after a transfer. There should be no gaps in knowledgeable oversight. The opportunity to obtain palliation advice at any time (24 hours a day and 7 days a week, if practicable) is greatly valued by patients and families. It will help limit readmissions to hospital from home or from a care institution when there is worry over some change in condition or comfort.

Of the several sites where a patient with advanced neurological disorder may receive care, an *aged or chronic care facility* is probably where most care must be managed. Continuing care in the *acute hospital* setting is usually inappropriate because of cost and the need to provide beds for other acute-care patients. Placement in a specialized in-patient *hospice* for terminal illness is unlikely to be available. Criteria regarding eligibility for admission to each category of care site (hospital, nursing home, residential care) vary

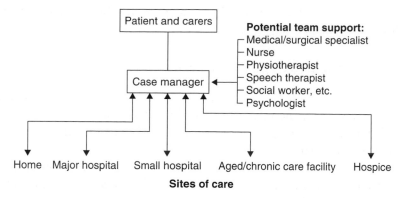

Figure 1.2.1   The many sites of care to which a patient may be directed; coordination of various supports at various places by one manager.

from country to country and from time to time, and insurance payments or government allocations may be limited in arbitrary ways. At various times in the long course of a neurological illness, the patient may shift between hospital and home, or between aged care or nursing home facility and hospital. It is desirable that one team, or at least one case manager from within a multi-disciplinary team remains available to the patient and family throughout these transitions, ensuring good communication and continuity of management (Figure 1.2.1).

IT RELIES ON TEAMWORK AND NETWORKING

No single individual can provide care that satisfies fully the principles of palliative management. The *multi-disciplinary team* is the preferred provider of palliation for neurological disease. Each member of the team brings a particular expertise that complements what is provided by others, and shares that contribution at regular team meetings, following the changing needs of the patient and becoming involved as and when that expertise is required.

Networking is a process of reaching out beyond the activity of that team to call upon the expertise, guidance or encouragement of related professional individuals, teams or institutions for the benefit of that same population of need.

It may often be the case that a well-structured team is available in one site of care (possibly major hospital or community setting) but it has no responsibility to continue care in another site, an aged care facility or a small hospital or another community. Every effort should be made in planning an individual's care to ensure that, through networking, the fullest possible range of disciplines remain available throughout the illness.

IT ADJUSTS ITS APPROACH IN RECOGNITION OF DETERIORATION

What medications can now be ceased? Drugs prescribed to lower cholesterol, to reduce blood pressure or prevent gout may be considered unnecessary and ceased in many cases. Is there really a need to keep encouraging the patient to perform activity that is daily more difficult? The patient should have permission to decide, and will often prefer to rest, focusing on the preservation of strength and action for preferred times such as receiving valued visitors.

The same approach can extend to common investigations (blood tests and X-rays). Unless a change in management will be guided by the result of an investigation, it ought not be requested. Even routine nursing observations (blood pressure, pulse and temperature readings) may be no longer useful, and can be replaced by regular symptom score assessments. Patients, family members or staff can be encouraged to assess specific discomforts on a daily (or more or less frequent) basis, giving a score (of, say, 0–10) for each common discomfort such as pain, nausea, anxiety or fatigue, and recording this so that progression can be noted, and symptoms recognized and managed promptly (see p. 35).

A particular worry for family members may be the patient's increasing disinterest in food. They may want to force food on the patient, and despair when their efforts meet resistance. It is usually more appropriate to allow the patient to indicate what food and how much is taken.

IT INCLUDES BEREAVEMENT SUPPORT

Concern for family members properly extends into the time after death, arranging bereavement support for those who were strongly affected by the loss of a loved one. Neurology staff members who have been associated with the patient over a long period will be warmly welcomed if they accept a role also in bereavement support. The period of anticipating loss is often as significant and stressful as the actual final event. Bereavement support begins, therefore, with the close relationships established with both patient and family members during the period of care. It includes honest reflections on the reality of what is happening, gentle exploration of thoughts and feelings, or plans for the time which will come after the time of caring has passed.

Some family caregivers will have abandoned employment in order to offer constant care over a prolonged period. After many years of dedicated supportive care they are now 'free', but how readily are they able to make use of that freedom; what new meaning can they give to life?

There is very little evidence that any particular bereavement intervention makes a significant difference to outcome. Palliative care experience suggests, however, that a follow-up letter or phone call, a visit and the offer of participation in a bereavement programme or group when there is any indication of a difficult bereavement, is highly valued. If staff who were involved in care during the terminal period can be available to participate, their contribution will be particularly appreciated (see pp. 118–119).

3

Nodal points in decision-making

INTRODUCING A PALLIATIVE MANAGEMENT APPROACH
(Figure 1.3.1, Point 1)

For incurable neurological diseases, palliative management offers an amelioration of discomfort, an avoidance of complications and a possible extension of life. It should be emphasized, however, that the diagnosis of an 'obstinate' or incurable condition must be firmly established before introducing patient and family to palliative or end stage care.

Once the clinical situation is clear, it is desirable that patient and family be introduced to its reality soon after diagnosis, along with a clear exposition of what can be done to maintain the best possible quality of life. Far from offering a message that 'nothing can be done', the neurologist tries to provide a positive view of the many supports that can help make life worthwhile. That is the essence of palliation.

The clinician may sketch out a *future clinical pathway*, sometimes called *a coordinated care plan*, one that emphasizes the several contributions to care that will be desirable or essential to ensure comfort and best possible function. The future clinical pathway will consider these components:

- Therapies that can slow or modify unwelcome changes and assist function.
- Site(s) of care that will best suit the patient and family.
- A list of the persons who can assist in care, their roles and contact details.
- Equipment appropriate to patient need, site and carer abilities.
- Information and training in knowledge and skills needed by carers.
- Medications that may reduce discomforts.
- Support services that help maintain independence and function, and how to access them.

- Access to 24-h advice for patient or family, usually by telephone.
- Access to emotional and spiritual support.
- A programme for regular review, to assess progress, monitor and respond to change.

A coordinated care plan may then be drawn up, and list the following:

- Observations that can be ceased as unnecessary.
- Drugs that can be discontinued.
- Pharmaceutical options for ensuring best level of comfort.
- A program of allied health interventions to assist and maintain function.
- Site of care options and when review should be made.
- Education opportunities for family members to enhance care skills and understanding.
- Information about who to call for help and under what circumstances.
- The timing and frequency of support available from doctor, nurse, equipment supplier, pastoral care worker, physiotherapist, etc.

Cognitive dysfunction and failure often occurs early in the course of a neurological disease, and the plan may include the writing of an advance directive, or the nomination of a proxy decision-maker for a future when the patient may become unable to make an informed decision (see chapters on Advance Directives and Proxy Decision-Making in Section IV, p. 201).

INTRODUCING PALLIATIVE INTERVENTIONS
(Figure 1.3.1, Points 2)

Some palliative interventions will have been required from the start of the illness, and been arranged by the attending neurology team. They may have called on the assistance of surgeons, other specialists and allied health professionals. At certain points in the progress of the illness there may also be advantage in recruiting, for a particular situation, the skills of one or other members of a palliative care team. This will depend primarily, of course, on whether such

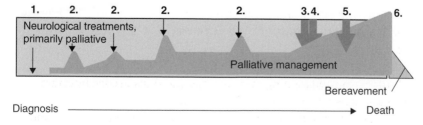

Figure 1.3.1 Decision points in the progress of a neurological condition.

individuals are available. The advantage of their involvement is that they may be more accustomed to planning with patients and families the final life journey. They can sometimes help patients face the disappointments of further deterioration and grave prognosis by bringing a sensitive understanding of the emotional and spiritual associations of such disappointments, and be able to offer some useful practical advice on how to maintain comfort and function.

TIMING THE ONSET OF THE TERMINAL PHASE
(Figure 1.3.1, Point 3)

Further along in the course of the illness, attending staff will begin to recognize that serious deterioration seems inevitable, signalling the onset of a terminal phase. The closer approach of death will be heralded by markers that may not be very obvious, because the patient often is unable to describe changing discomforts, and the disease progression may be subtle and gradual. A team decision, drawing upon the reflections of patient, family, intimate carers, attending staff and specialist physician, may be helpful in determining the onset of the terminal phase.

Speaking openly about such a transition is always difficult. Hopes for some improvement or delay in the decline of function remain, and these are natural mechanisms for coping with the disappointments of advanced and progressive illness. For many persons affected by neurological conditions, the long-standing emphasis of supportive care has been on maintaining strength and independence. Now comes a time when it may be a better course to cease striving for function, and focus on whatever brings pleasure or relief, aiming to make the best of the acknowledged short time that is left, rather than seek after some greater length of days at all costs.

Careful discussion with patient and family should be undertaken to achieve a common understanding, and to receive permission for appropriate changes in the approach to care: for example, to stop an expensive drug which is bringing little or no benefit, to resign from the effort of daily physiotherapy, to place the emphasis now on comfort and to stop the desperate struggle to provide a daily demonstration of courage and patience; and even (perhaps) to cease life-supporting ventilation.*

---

*Worldwide, there is great variation in the way in which refusal or withdrawal of treatment is considered. In those countries where palliative care services have been long established, there is commonly a strong support for patient decision-making, and for the patient's right to request cessation of treatment, even when this is regarded as maintaining life. In other countries, it is regarded as improper or illegal to cease a treatment that is maintaining life, even when that treatment is uncomfortable and is being continued against the patient's expressed wish.

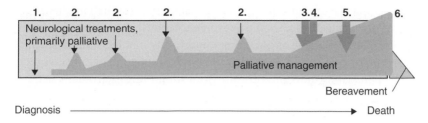

Figure 1.3.1 Decision points in the progress of a neurological condition.

REFERRAL TO A PALLIATIVE CARE TEAM (Figure 1.3.1, Point 4)

If it is available, the support of a palliative care team may be recruited. The family may have already met members of such a service when particular palliative interventions were suggested earlier in the course of the illness. Palliative care staff are comfortable in assisting patients and families to face the reality of continuing deterioration and eventual death. Referral to a palliative care service often signifies more clearly to patient and family the reality of approaching death, and it also indicates an intention to make the final journey as satisfactorily as possible.

Such a referral should not indicate that the neurology team is abandoning any interest and involvement in the process of care. Sharing and coordination will be most helpful, allowing a gradual shift in responsibility. Sometimes, referral to a palliative care team will be resisted as 'negative' thinking by both families and professionals. They will be unwilling to accept the reality of deterioration, and will reject such a referral, even in the very last days of life. In that case, the neurology team must continue to carry the full responsibility for palliative management.

WRITING A 'DO NOT RESUSCITATE' ORDER (Figure 1.3.1, Point 5)

Sometimes the recognition of whether the terminal phase has been approached will be highlighted by a request (by nursing staff or ambulance staff) to indicate whether a *'do not resuscitate'* (DNR) order applies. Ideally this should be discussed with the patient and the family, as well as other involved staff. Usually the decision that active resuscitation would be inappropriate is well accepted, particularly if it can be framed in positive terms, that the approach now is focused on good palliative management, and the avoidance of intrusions that are potentially uncomfortable and unlikely to alter the course of the disease (Figure 1.3.1).

The practice of undertaking cardiopulmonary resuscitation after death from a non-acute disease should be avoided. Even when resuscitation is performed (and defended) as a training opportunity in a teaching hospital, it shows no respect for the deceased, and distracts attending family members from appreciating the reality of death, from supporting each other's sadness and grief, and from making such arrangements as are necessary to inform wider family members and friends, and plan funeral arrangements together.

Rephrasing the 'DNR' instruction as a 'good palliative care' order, a positive intention to focus on comfort rather than length of days, has won wide approval.

INTRODUCING BEREAVEMENT CARE (Figure 1.3.1, Points 3–6)

Palliative care programmes in many countries have pioneered bereavement support for family members and close friends of individuals who have died from cancer. This has been taken up in some other situations, for example in accident and emergency rooms where sudden unexpected death is a relatively common event, and grief for survivors may be intense.

Death coming at the end of a long and distressing illness, and often in an old person, may not appear to arouse a similar intensity of grief. But a family will often feel that they have suffered a succession of losses, as mental and physical functions in the affected individual decay progressively, causing a serial sense of bereavement. Often, there has been a long time of commitment to care, and the fact that some neurological patients are quite young (e.g. muscular dystrophy) can mean a very real loss of meaning and an emptiness in the lives of carers after death has occurred. It may help if bereavement support has already started earlier in the course of the illness, but other particular supports may be valued after death has occurred (see pp. 118–119).

None of these suggested nodal occasions for decision-making should be seen as single points in time; each one, but particularly the introduction of the reality of the terminal phase, and the involvement of a palliative care team, may be mentioned tentatively, and returned to over a period of time, waiting for a fuller awareness to be accepted, and a decision quietly reached.

4

Common deficiencies in palliative management

POOR COMMUNICATION

Communication is a two-way process, and liable to be inhibited by factors that limit the ability of either party to enter into a full and free exchange. In the acute in-patient setting a clinician's communications are usually clearly directed and brief, focused on immediate problems and providing crisp management strategies and prescriptions. When the patient response is inhibited or slowed by changes in *appreciation* (as in dementia, deafness or delirium) or in *expression* (as in a large number of neurodegenerative conditions) there is a temptation for attending persons to be impatient, to guess at need, to assume permission for new interventions, to accept a role of speaking at the patient rather than exchanging with the patient. It is always worth remembering that impairment that creates difficulty or inability to communicate does not necessarily indicate a lack of awareness or understanding.

Impaired communication may originate from focal cerebral lesions, causing:

- *aphasia*: an inability to cope with both the reception and expression of information;
- *agnosia*: a failure to give meaning to stimuli which are received; or
- *apraxia*: a disturbance of voluntary intent in movement (in this case of the muscles serving speech), so that some automatic responses may come through, but the processing of thought into action is impaired.

Dysarthria, and paresis affecting respiration, laryngeal function or movements of the tongue, palate or lips will inhibit expression even when there may be clarity of thought. Confusion may result from metabolic changes, medication side-effects, and numerous other causes.

In seeking *consent*, whether for starting or ceasing a treatment, or considering transfer to another site of care, adequate communication with the patient is essential. Effective communication calls for patience, and deliberate involvement of family members who have a close familiarity with the patient and who can assist with providing information in ways that the patient can understand, and in interpreting what the patient says.

It will always be appropriate to make a consistent effort to speak as directly as possible to the patient, and to avoid focusing only on a proxy informant (family or staff member), even when the patient retains little or no capacity for exchange.

An individual who has lost virtually all power to hear or understand the spoken word or who is unable to communicate with speech, already feels marginalized, discounted and excluded. Face-to-face confrontation, touch and gesture may yet convey or elicit some element of meaningful communication.

Communication aids

The services of a speech therapist able to call upon specialized techniques and access electronic aids/appliances that can increase choice and independence for severely disabled people will be of great value in particular cases. Electronic assistive technology (also called environmental control equipment) is increasingly sophisticated and affordable. Even where movement is limited to the eyelids or eye muscles, it may be possible to establish a reliable call mechanism, a set of signals to indicate specific decisions and choices, or even a means for spelling out quite detailed messages. The assurance of control that such aids can provide is of immense importance to a severely disabled individual.

What to say

Apart from the difficulties that may block effective exchange between physician and patient, there is the issue of what is to be the desired *content* of that exchange. In working with persons affected by advanced neurological disorders and with their families there are few opportunities for conveying good news. Most news will be bad or sad, and difficult to express. As the process of evolution and deterioration in many such diseases is relatively slow, health care staff will often regard stages of decline as inevitable, 'only to be expected', and may fail to take full account of the consequences for home life, social activity, sexual expression, work or sense of self-worth that are impacting on the patient and the family members.

There is a tendency to discount the opinions, preferences and directions of individuals who are experiencing the advanced stage of an incurable illness. Elderly persons housed in institutional settings in Western societies frequently complain that the staff speak to them as though they were children. In the same way those seeking to support individuals in the terminal stage of an illness may judge that the effects of the disease, the medications, the unfamiliar surroundings or the threat of imminent death are disturbing cognition and the ability to make appropriate decisions, and therefore make little or no attempt to communicate with them.

Part of the task of palliation can be to gently encourage both family and staff to make renewed attempts to understand and consider what the patient's wishes are. Perhaps the patient is stating a clear request that family members cannot accept; for example, to die quickly, or (in quite different mode) to undertake heroic interventions that family and attending physicians see as expensive, quite inappropriate and probably fatal. The patient may refuse absolutely to leave home and receive care in an appropriate facility, when that is the recommendation of the physician and the hope of the family.

Such requests and refusals need to be heard with patience and affection, and, where possible, turned gently towards what is reasonable, on common-sense grounds, legally allowed, technically feasible and medically justifiable.

General principles

For many individuals, communication with a person facing advanced and terminal illness is a source of considerable stress. 'I do not know what to say', is a common feeling, particularly when the discussion must centre on the clinical reality and the communication of bad news. Buckman, a Canadian physician, has emphasized some of the components that are generally important in facilitating such discussions. They include consideration of the setting for the discussion, which should offer quiet and comfort, and allow eye contact and touch (if able to be offered naturally and appropriately). The professional must try to convey an undivided attention and an absence of hurry.

The purpose of the interview and the role of the interviewer are first made clear. Others who may be present (family, staff) need to be acknowledged and welcomed. Listening is the basic skill to be used. Silences should be tolerated. One person skilled in exchange with persons suffering advanced cancer has written, '*Most of my talk was in silence; but that has been the only worthwhile talk of my life*'. Open questions which invite a patient response are best, and meeting that response with a nod or a 'hmmm' or the repetition of a phrase spoken by the patient will be helpful. To clarify uncertainties, one can ask: 'When you said that, did you mean ... ?'

A further important step will be to acknowledge the feelings that the patient or family member seems to be expressing. 'It must have been difficult for you ...' 'That might have made you quite angry?' Feelings are valid; there is no place for discounting or judging them.

Bad news

When it comes to the giving of bad news, it will be helpful if some forewarning has been conveyed earlier. If tests have been ordered, it may have been possible to indicate that the results may have either good or not so good implications. To convey bad news demands that permission has been given to share whatever needs to be said. Sometimes it may be necessary to ask, 'How much do you want to know at this stage?', recognizing that a patient has a right to know and a right also not to know. In that case, one may ask if it is preferred that a family member should be given fuller information. It is often very helpful (some might say, essential) to have another person, a friend or relative, sharing in the interview when bad news has to be mentioned.

Given permission, it is important to say enough, but not too much, using simple terms to convey the facts as known, and checking what has been heard and understood. As well as checking that the information has been received, it is important to be ready to acknowledge the emotional response to the information, offering, perhaps an empathetic opener such as 'This must be not what you hoped for', or 'This has been hard for me to talk about; it must be much harder for you'.

Bad news in the supportive phase

A person with advanced and potentially terminal disease faces a succession of bad news announcements. There is the time of diagnosis, when distress may be lightened by the offer of some therapies able to restore comfort, at least for a time. But then discomforts and disabilities recur, and the failure to achieve hoped-for outcomes must be acknowledged. Finally there will be questions about how long a survival may be expected, and what the terminal phase will be like. As such information cannot be accurate in its predictions, vague responses may cause additional stress. In degenerative diseases, where the pace of decline is slow and variable, uncertainties can continue over a long time, and living with uncertainty is not easy.

Bad news in the terminal phase

The terminal phase of the illness often may be complicated by impaired cognition or by major physical or emotional disabilities making communication particularly difficult, and that will direct the emphasis in communication towards close relatives or friends. But every effort should be made to maintain a therapeutic exchange directly with the patient.

It is usually better that bad news is conveyed rather than deliberately withheld. The way in which bad news is told, however, is as important as its factual content.

It is rarely helpful to tell an untruth, or to pretend that the situation is better than it really is. Even when what needs to be said seems certain to cause great sorrow or emotional pain, it should be made clear. *But not immediately, or all at once.* A truthful response to a question or a new offer of information can be the opportunity to offer a small preliminary warning of the possibility of bad news. It can be said, for example, that perhaps as the patient's situation becomes clearer (whether with a further test or the passage of time) one possible result will be quite bad news. Some time later, a further examination or test confirms what was mentioned as possible, and the reality of the situation can be more fully outlined.

The timing, site, choice of words, and who is to be present will all need consideration. The conveying of information is a process, not accomplished in a single conversation; something returned to, perhaps in a less formal context following from a conversation about other happier things of interest to the patient and the family.

RIGID PROFESSIONAL BOUNDARIES

It is common in medical practice everywhere for physicians to be protective of the relationship they have established with their patients, and to feel reluctant to refer patients to other physicians for opinion or for further care, except where other specialist assistance is clearly necessary. The reasons for such reluctance are possibly many, but may include protection of income, a determination to appear effective and able to manage more than a narrow range of expertise, or a dependence on the admiration offered by the patient. Feeling a need to defend one's own field of operation is a frequent human attribute; establishing a clear boundary between the area of one's own expertise and that of other workers often seems attractive. As the American poet Robert Frost suggests in a well-known poem ('*Mending Wall*'): 'Good fences make good neighbours'; when we acknowledge each other's area of ownership and respect it, we are comfortable with one another.

In providing palliation to an individual with advanced illness, however, there is a need to *transcend established boundaries*, and build respect within open cooperation. An ideal arrangement is often 'shared care', with physicians interested in active treatment of disease working alongside those who are concerned with ensuring comprehensive patient comfort and dignity. Other medical and surgical specialties may have important interventions to offer, but also spiritual and pastoral advisers, nursing colleagues, allied health workers.

When the human need of the patient is the central concern, the professional standing assumed by the attending physician must take second place to a humble recognition that it is with the help of a cooperating team that the well-being of the patient will be best assured.

INEFFECTIVE NETWORKING

There are two complementary aspects of networking:

(a) Being aware of, and being comfortable with, the value of assistance from the many disciplines and skills that are available in the wider world of health care, and being ready to invite their cooperation in the management of an individual.

(b) Being available to assist colleagues from other disciplines and institutions with advice, opinion and support of the care they offer.

The range of potential contributors to a palliative management network is wide. Many neurologists will be used to seeking the advice of other specialist physicians, but they may be less used to working alongside family doctors, hospital nurses (who increasingly command specialist skills), community nurses, physiotherapists, speech therapists, psychologists, aged care workers, volunteers, community support organizations, priests and pastoral care workers.

There are sub-specialties in neurology that any professional outside of that particular focus of expertise should feel ready to approach for advice and assistance. Examples may include the management of difficult cases of epilepsy or Parkinson's disease, or the use of botulinum toxin or of intrathecal pumps to deliver baclofen or analgesia.

Palliative management that continues through to the time of death needs a comprehensive management plan (see p. 20), in which the various components of care are recruited for their particular contributions at the best times and in the appropriate places. Such a plan needs a focus or a leader who is able to draw in, when they are required, the various resources that will make the plan work satisfactorily. A neurologist who has become familiar with this approach to palliation will often be well placed to provide that leadership, or to offer clinical support to an internist or family physician who assumes that role. In all clinical care for a needy patient there is a temptation for the provider of care to assume a strong sense of responsibility, but that should not lead to a feeling of 'ownership', or reluctance to recognize the benefit of other specialist advice or intervention.

POORLY DEVELOPED TEAMWORK

Where continuing care proves inadequate, it will often be found to be due to the lack of both teamwork and networking. Teamwork implies a group of professionals (and volunteers also, where possible) who acknowledge a common loyalty to an institution or programme and a common commitment to a process of care for persons with particular needs. Their involvement is iterative, following the changing needs of the patient and providing appropriate expertise as and when it is required.

Teamwork and networking usually have been better understood and implemented in palliative care and in geriatric and rehabilitation medicine than in neurology. A critical characteristic of teamwork is mutual understanding and respect between individual team members. It will be common (but not essential) for a physician to be recognized as the leader of the team. That should not result, however, in a hierarchical structure that either leads non-medical members of the team to show undue deference to their leader, or makes it difficult for the leader to listen to, and be advised by, the experience and skills of the other members of the team.

In long-term neurological care there can be a problem in the setting and acceptance of common goals for care *that derive from the patient*. A 'team' whose members set their own goals or have goals set for them by external agencies risks being dysfunctional if the agreed role is not one of elucidating the patient's need and formulating plans to meet that need.

Evaluation and intervention by a physiotherapist or masseur, a speech pathologist, a neuropsychologist or an occupational therapist may recommend some new procedures or the introduction of regular activities that general staff or family can take up and use in promoting greater physical and emotional comfort. A social worker may help lift some of the burden of care from a family by arranging respite support or financial assistance. A pastoral care worker or trained volunteer may contribute through an awareness of patient fears and hopes, and non-judgemental listening. The availability and practised use of communication aids, mobility aids and other appropriate equipment of good quality suggested by an occupational therapist can make a major difference to the morale of both patients and their carers.

It will be equally important to be ready to decide when to *cease* certain interventions.

In established guidelines for the management of stroke, for example, referral to expert opinion is recommended for guidance on:

- swallowing or communication difficulties (speech therapist);
- nutrition (nutritionist);
- mobility limitations (physiotherapist);
- impairment of activities of daily living (occupational therapist);
- perceptual difficulties (neuropsychologist);
- incontinence (continence nurse).

Such specialists are not always quick to detect abnormalities in areas that lie outside their own specific area of expertise. As the various disabilities and discomforts continue, and possibly worsen, therefore, it may be time for a more global assessment by a single physician with the assistance of one or two nurses who have known the patient intimately over a period of time.

FAILURE TO MAINTAIN AN ACCESSIBLE CLINICAL RECORD

A *written record* is the basic tool of health care communication. Whether it is prepared and stored electronically or on paper, the clinical record should be able to be accessed easily by all those who contribute to management.

Often, the best place to store such a running record of the work of the many potential contributors to care is close to the patient. This happens in a hospital, where clinical notes and treatment sheets are held at the ward desk. For home care, a *patient-held record*, or agreement to keep case-notes *in the home*, may be best. In the home setting, as in the hospital or other institution it will be most useful if *all persons* involved in care (even volunteers) are encouraged to record their contributions in the case-notes. Teamwork and networking are facilitated when individual contributions to care, at whatever site, are recorded in ways that can be accessed by other care providers.

5

Common themes in palliation practice

There are common themes within palliation practice that have relevance to many of the diseases under consideration and the common discomforts that are experienced:

1. *Holism*: considering multiple interactions and influences.
2. *Recording observations of distress*: analogue scales.
3. *Involving the team*: communicating, recording and supporting.
4. *No correct answer*: innovation and experiment.
5. *Appropriate therapy regimens.*
6. *Support of carers.*
7. *Working with complementary and alternative medicine.*

HOLISM

Holism was a term coined by the South African philosopher and statesman Jan Christian Smuts. It signifies that an entity is more than the sum of its parts, that it will not be fully understood by analysis, but will also need an appreciation of its operation as a whole, and the many relationships that bear upon it.

The term has been well received by practitioners of palliation, who recognize that disability, discomfort and dependency (common outcomes of neurological disease) create a complex pattern of distress that is not satisfactorily described as a list of symptoms, but needs also an awareness of the way daily life of the affected individual has been changed in its physical, emotional and spiritual components. Spiritual and emotional needs are just as real as physical ones, and may need to be approached by persons drawn from outside the conventional medical scene. These may be clergy, priests, imams or monks from one or another religious faith, but may equally be individuals sufficiently confident in their own understanding of 'spirit' to open discussion and listen to the questions of another.

Holism also implies a recognition that symptoms interact; that nausea, for example, makes pain worse, that constipation affects comfort in many dimensions. Some of the common discomforts of neurological disease attract little medical interest either because they are not readily amenable to improvement, or because they are difficult to characterize or measure. Fatigue, weakness, stiffness, thirst, sadness, difficulty in finding a comfortable resting posture, a poor appetite, a dry mouth and alteration in taste or ability to smell – any of these may erode total comfort quite markedly, but readily escape the attention of a busy clinician.

RECORDING OF OBSERVATIONS

Recording distress therefore needs both a global measure and individual attention to a list of common symptoms that includes those often missed as well as the more dramatic and treatable ones. The search for a satisfactory global measure of quality of life has proved quite difficult. Some attempts have involved complex questionnaires charting responses to many aspects of life. Others depend on one simple question. Balfour Mount, a leading Canadian palliative care pioneer has suggested the double question, 'How are you?' (often met with a cheerful or optimistic response, as we do in everyday life), followed by, 'How are you in yourself?' may sometimes bring out a more revealing comment.

The recording of symptoms is, when dealing with the terminal phase of an illness, of greater interest and significance than are the usual routine observations commonly made in hospital practice (temperature, pulse, respiration or blood pressure). Sometimes, when a nurse reports an unusually low blood pressure in a wasted bed-bound individual, the appropriate response may be 'Stop taking it'.

Patients and their carers quickly learn to use a simple analogue scale to report the intensity of important symptoms: 0–10 or (more simple and probably just as satisfactory) 0–5; 0 being no discomfort at all related to that particular symptom and the upper number, 5 or 10, representing the very worst discomfort it can be imagined to cause. Recording, in this way, particular symptoms that are known to be important to the patient, will chart changes and the usefulness of measures taken to reduce their impact (Figure 1.5.1).

DATE

SYMPTOM	scale	3/4	4/4	5/4	6/4	7/4	8/4	9/4	10/4	11/4	12/4
PAIN	5										
	4										
	3										
	2										
	1										
	0										
FATIGUE	5										
	4										
	3										
	2										
	1										
	0										
DRY MOUTH	5										
	4										
	3										
	2										
	1										
	0										
POOR SLEEP	5										
	4										
	3										
	2										
	1										
	0										

Figure 1.5.1   Daily record of symptoms. (Adapted from Bruera *et al. Journal of Palliative Care* 1991; 7(2): 6–9.) (See reference p. 236.)

Analogue scales to rate the intensity of selected symptoms day-by-day (or more frequently if required) are often employed. This example uses a scale of 0–5; attending staff are encouraged to colour in the squares to a number that represents the patient's, or their own, judgement of the degree of discomfort (see reference: Bruera *et al*. The Edmonton symptom assessment system (ESAS) scale).

In the above example, pain is shown to have been quickly controlled over the first 3 days, but fatigue has become more of a problem, dry mouth has been difficult to relieve satisfactorily and poor sleep is very variable and intermittent. Various persons who are attending the patient can contribute to the visual record being produced, and a quick glance at the record reveals how effectively discomforts are being dealt with.

These are symptoms that matter to the patient. By charting them and displaying them routinely at change-over times and team meetings, or by having the family chart them for the next visit of the nurse or doctor, there is a clear picture of the common components of discomfort, helping to focus care on what may help the patient best.

FINDING THE BEST ANSWER: INNOVATION AND EXPERIMENT

As palliative management is guided by the response of the patient, and because of the subjective and very variable nature of symptoms and how they are experienced, it is often quite impossible to set clear guidelines for management or to be confident that a particular intervention will be effective.

This is well illustrated in the use of analgesics. There is no 'correct' dose for an opioid. Some individuals will have their pain eliminated with a tiny dose (oral morphine 2.5 mg), others will need much larger doses to gain any relief at all. Some patients will become confused and delirious on a small dose of one opioid, or suffer distressing nausea, but tolerate another opioid with no difficulty. One patient will receive great relief from physiotherapy; another with an apparently similar musculo-skeletal symptom feel worse. The clinician therefore needs to start small, to regard every intervention and prescription as an experiment, and to be ready to follow-up promptly, and make changes when necessary.

APPROPRIATE THERAPY REGIMENS

Ceasing unnecessary medications
Some medications prescribed in the supportive phase of care will remain relevant and effective in the later stages, but often it will be possible to cease others; for example, for cardiovascular conditions (hypertension, hyperlipidaemia, cardiac ischaemia) or arthritis (the patient now becoming immobile). If swallowing becomes difficult, attempts to take oral tablets and capsules can be a source of additional discomfort.

Administration of medications when swallowing is difficult
In the presence of weakness and dysphagia, the route for drug administration will commonly need re-assessment. The subcutaneous (S/C) route is usually more convenient than intravenous (I-V) infusion, and more acceptable and more predictable than rectal administration. Many relevant drugs can be used via S/C infusion or bolus injection, and there are several models of portable battery-powered infusion pumps that deliver continuous infusions very precisely over 24 h. The list of drugs suitable to infuse in this way includes:

- *Analgesics*: opioids – morphine, hydromorphone, fentanyl, oxycodone, diamorphine (whichever is available); ketamine, clonidine, lignocaine (for neuropathic or difficult pain).

- *Anti-emetics*: metoclopramide, haloperidol, ondansetron and other 5HT3 antagonists.
- *Anticonvulsant*: clonazepam.
- *Sedatives*: midazolam.
- *Antispasmodics*: baclofen, hyoscine butylbromide.
- *Anticholinergics*: hyoscine hydrobromide.

Many of these medications can be combined in a single infusion, but some combinations are not appropriate, either because of drug interaction or precipitation in the syringe (e.g. dexamethasone together with midazolam causes a clouding of the solution).

All of the above medications can also be administered I-V.

Some parenteral medications are better administered by bolus injection:

- *S/C*: dexamethasone, phenobarbitone.
- *Deep intramuscular (I-M) injection*: chlorpromazine, diazepam.
- *I-V*: phenytoin.

SUPPORT OF CARERS

The progressive loss of function and increasing difficulty with communication put a strain on relationships. Family members may not be able to cope with the prospect of many years spent as a carer rather than spouse or lover, employers have little capacity to continue the employment of a family breadwinner who is now partly disabled, or of a full time carer.

Practical help

A comprehensive care programme will include some attention to simple practical measures that make life more possible for family members and carers undertaking home care. These may include financial assistance for the purchase of drugs, dressings and disposables. In some situations health care is free but social care is limited (e.g. by a means test). Complex care for an illness may therefore be much more readily accessed than is basic domestic support. Family members need to know what home nursing and allied health assistance they can call upon, what equipment will make care easier, and how it is obtained; and what assistance with domestic tasks such as cleaning or preparing meals can be arranged. Volunteer assistance for sitting with the patient while carers have time to shop or visit away from the home is usually much valued.

Education

Inclusion of the patient and of family members in preparing a comprehensive plan of management is a central feature of home care. Each of the major progressive neurological diseases has special features, but in nearly all of them there are fears and frustrations common to patients and carers alike. Simple information about the particular disease they confront, written in easily understood ways, is a basic step. It will not be a litany of bad news, but focus on offering practical suggestions for how family can assist the patient in making the most of limited function and maintaining a sense of control in a deteriorating situation. What is ahead for them? What should they expect, be prepared for?

Respite

Where family and friends continue to provide the major part of care and support they themselves rarely receive the support they need in their own right: depression is common and stress levels are high. Those directly providing care will almost certainly have had to give up their own job and social life; they too will be isolated. Respite care, which could enable them to maintain some social contact and retain some outside interests and thus ease their burden greatly, is hard to come by, its lack of availability compounded by lack of funding. The burden of care for an individual with advanced neurological degenerative disease can lead to carer exhaustion and burnout. Opportunity for short periods of holiday and recuperation by arranging a brief admission of the patient to an appropriate institution may restore carer energy and motivation. In larger centres the different needs of younger patient age groups may be met with special activities such as weekend retreats. These have proved valuable for patients (and their carers) coping with muscular dystrophy, amyotrophic lateral sclerosis (ALS), Parkinson's disease or multiple sclerosis (MS).

Advocacy

In some countries the division of responsibility for care between health and social care leads to further conflict and damage to self-esteem. This conflict is even more marked when health care is provided free of charge but social care is means tested (as for example, in the UK). Arbitrary decisions that protect budgets but deny people much needed assistance create additional obstacles.

There is a need for professionals involved in care for this group of people to listen to their experiences and to make use of what they hear in formulating representations to professional bodies, local authorities and government.

Whether in palliative care or neurology, we are not free from blame for our failure to advocate for better support of people in the late stages of neurological conditions.

Emotional support

The frustrations of impaired function are compounded for many patients by the feeling of being a burden. The intensity of that burden falls largely on close family members. The course of the disease may be inexorable (as with ALS) or variable (as with MS); in either case there is uncertainty, inhibition of future plans for family members, erosion of financial resources and the introduction of new tensions into family dynamics. Opportunity for carers to express their frustrations and troubles is helpful, and sometimes it may be very useful to suggest a family meeting where the way care is being conducted and how it is affecting family members can be openly discussed, with, hopefully, agreement reached about any changes to routines.

In many centres there are community groups formed around the needs of those with a particular disease. They aim to support carers, to advocate for resources of potential benefit, and facilitate access to them by integrating them into a cooperating service able to address all aspects of a care situation. Mutual support groups encourage self-help and promote positivity and hope. Web sites have been established all around the world, helping access to authoritative information (but also some of dubious authority!) and offering a global opportunity for sharing.

Carer fatigue and burnout

It is not uncommon for family members to experience compassion and support fatigue after long months and years of providing home care or undertaking regular visits to an institution. When a patient who previously was an active participant in family affairs slowly deteriorates to a point where there can be little or no meaningful exchange, tired family members may see little point in the continuing responsibility for daily care or the regular visits to the care facility. A wish for the illness to take its course quickly is understandable, but is often difficult to express, and may arouse feelings of anger or guilt. Where appropriate, warm applause for the support that has been provided over a long time is helpful, and open discussion about the present situation is usually welcomed, together with clarification of what can be said concerning prognosis and terminal symptoms. There must be time for questions and reflections, some of which will not come easily. The opportunity for discussion and support prior to death is an important contribution to bereavement care.

Bereavement care

Families that have remained together throughout such a devastating and demeaning journey as care for a person with a chronic neurological condition can be, deserve admiration and respect. When the final stages arrive they will have much to offer but will, themselves, also have great need. Feelings of guilt, of anger, of relief and of grief will be mixed together. They should be given time to talk through some of their feelings in an environment that allows expressions of anger without fear of criticism. After the death, after years devoted to caring, they will need help to find a new purpose in life at a time when their conflicting emotions continue to make it difficult for them to adjust.

Sudden and unanticipated death presents the greatest difficulty for those bereaved by loss. In the setting of deterioration from neurological disease, there will often have been a long time of anticipation and then a succession of losses: loss of strength, mobility, voice, clarity of mind, responsive presence. There may be a warm breathing body, but the personality of the one with terminal disease seems absent: '*I lost him years ago*'. Death comes, very often, as a relief and a release. But sadness, grief and its accompaniments of depression, distraction, sleeplessness, restlessness or anger may still supervene, and feelings of guilt can loom large as a cause of emotional difficulty. Simple follow-up mechanisms for checking on close family most affected by the loss remain important (see pp. 119–120).

WORKING ALONGSIDE COMPLEMENTARY AND ALTERNATIVE MEDICINE

In incurable progressive diseases that do not respond consistently to conventional therapies it is understandable that patients and family carers explore unconventional treatments. Desperate persons who hope for a cure by any means, however, risk being exploited by quacks and charlatans.

It is useful to separate complementary therapies from so-called 'alternative' treatments. Complementary treatments expand conventional treatments, offering interventions that are generally safe, gentle and pleasant, aimed at facilitating relaxation, comfort and confidence. They include massage and manipulation, hydrotherapy, aromatherapy, hypnosis and relaxation techniques. These are vehicles for palliation and ought usually to be welcomed as additions to care, providing extra measures of comfort for the patient.

Acupuncture, chiropractic, herbal therapies and homeopathy build on individual theories of disease causation and from these theories have evolved comprehensive systems of management. They are sustained by a long history of contributions to medical care and in practice are often used in complementary ways alongside conventional treatments.

There are many practitioners of alternative techniques, however, who make extravagant claims of cure founded in fanciful theory, and counsel their clients to avoid conventional treatments. Their alternative techniques include interventions such as colonic irrigation or enemas using various constituents ('to clear away toxins'), radical dietary regimens including controlled starvation, the use of magnetic attachments to the body and potions claiming a magical effect.

How should a clinician respond when patient or family demonstrate enormous faith in an alternative treatment that objective judgment finds to be lacking in credibility, and even potentially dangerous? It will be natural to feel irritation, even anger, particularly if the alternative treatment is very expensive and if its proponent disparages conventional approaches to care. Alternative practices sometimes carry an implied criticism of conventional medicine – it has been too negative, because seeing no prospect of cure it has become cursory and brief in the consultations, seeming to display a lack of interest. It is not appropriate to direct anger towards the patient or family, or even towards the alternative practitioner. First try to understand what attracts the family's confidence, what they have been promised.

If what is being offered as alternative therapy seems safe, perhaps there is no need to oppose it, but if it is possibly harmful, likely to cause unnecessary discomfort or complications, the clinician must reflect a concern – calmly, quietly and sensitively. It may help the family if an offer is made to explore further the technique being offered, to ascertain whether it has been recognized in reputable publications, or is known by colleagues. Sometimes (all too rarely!) there may be opportunity to contact the alternative practitioner and discuss the approach to management, in the hope that some mutual understanding can be reached. If the patient's situation is such that no conventional treatments seem to be helping, then alternative measures may be just as good or even better in supporting patient well-being.

Whatever is said or done, it should be left clear to the patient and family that the interest and support of the clinician and the clinical team remains available, and will continue to promote the highest standards of care and support.

SECTION II

Major Discomforts in Advanced Neurological Illness

Fatigue

Fatigue is 'a subjective lack of physical and/or mental energy that is perceived by the individual or caregiver to interfere with usual and desired activities'. It refers most appropriately to circumstances in which effort of any kind is exhausting, or is unable to be sustained for more than a short period.

A differential diagnosis of fatigue will endeavour to clarify contributory elements that are reversible, and will consider the following:

- relapse of disease,
- drug treatments,
- prolonged inactivity,
- cachexia,
- pain,
- anaemia,
- sleep disturbance,
- depressed mood,
- metabolic disorders,
- stress,
- fever.

Loss of energy and fatigue are major symptoms of depression, and may be helped by antidepressant medication (see Depression in Chapter 8 of this section, p. 114). Many drug treatments underlie persistent fatigue: anxiolytics, drugs for spasticity, anti-epileptics and interferon-beta. The correction of anaemia by blood transfusion or erythropoietin may improve well-being. The inflammatory reactions associated with solid cancers cause fatigue and may respond to corticosteroids with improved feelings of energy and capacity and a brighter mood.

Whereas weakness can be measured with simple assessments of muscle strength, fatigue, like pain, is a highly subjective discomfort, difficult to assess objectively and difficult to measure, though scales and symptom inventories have been devised which assist monitoring of progress, particularly in the one individual.

There are few specific therapies that lessen established fatigue:

- *caffeine 100 mg tab.* up to 4/day helps some individuals;
- *methylphenidate 10 mg tab.* 10–20 mg morning and midday offers some relief for drowsiness and mental fatigue but little to physical fatigue;
- *modafinil 100 mg tab.* 100–200 mg morning and noon or
- *amantadine 100 mg tab.* 100 mg once or twice daily in fatigue of multiple sclerosis have had some reported success, not supported by a systematic review;
- behaviour modification therapy and graded exercise have both been recommended, but lack high-level evidence of effectiveness.

An important part of the clinical approach to fatigue is the encouragement that can come from a realistic appraisal of the limitations imposed by the symptom and suggestions for making best use of whatever energy remains. Planned periods of rest, equipment to facilitate graded exercise, attention to stress reduction together with measures (drug and non-drug) for relief of anxiety and depression should be discussed. Any physical effort may seriously reduce subsequent energy. After a 'good day' that allowed an outing, the patient must expect additional fatigue, and should be allowed relief from enthusiastic encouragement to try again, and may need protection from all but the most necessary visitors. Companions who are able to provide the warmth of fellowship without making undue demands, and simple pleasures which can be enjoyed at rest – music, meditation, massage and conversation – should be explored as a part of clinical management. To let the patient be at rest, and provide a non-demanding presence that offers the gentle stimulus of reading, music or touch without expecting a response, is an important skill for family to learn.

2

Problems with muscles and movement

WEAKNESS

Muscle weakness has a multitude of causes. Some involve genetic or metabolic disturbances affecting the muscle directly, some are caused by interruptions to the transmission of impulses at the neuromuscular junction, still others by abnormalities in the muscle nerve supply. Disuse atrophy with profound weakness may be seen in advanced arthritis or in any other condition where chronic pain enforces immobility. There are numerous uncommon syndromes in which muscle weakness is an important component; many of these will come to a specialist neurologist for elucidation. Some weakness is temporary, recovery of strength often occurs in stroke or very commonly in Guillain–Barré syndrome. Cranial motor and peripheral muscular dysfunction in myasthenia gravis may respond to steroids, immuno-suppressants and either plasma exchange or immunoglobulin infusions as well as thymectomy and the use of pyridostigmine. There are presentations of 'functional' weakness (often unilateral and sometimes accompanied by sensory symptoms) commonly of prolonged duration, that are little altered by treatment of any kind, but are not readily assigned to any recognizable neurological diagnosis. This group of disorders reminds us that weakness is a subjective as well an objective and measurable symptom.

More pertinent to this discussion is the weakness, generalized or limited to particular muscle areas, that is associated with progressive neurological diseases such as amyotrophic lateral sclerosis (ALS), Parkinson's disease, multiple sclerosis (MS), the muscular dystrophies and neuropathies and with stroke and cerebral tumour.

The supportive phase
A disability or discomfort that is not amenable to treatment deserves palliation. But what is palliation for weakness? It comprises all those interventions that

enable an optimal continuity of physical function, whether by regular graded exercise; alterations in medication (e.g. reducing corticosteroid dose); supply of equipment to enhance mobility and substitute for diminished strength; or counselling to facilitate acceptance of an inevitable decline in power.

Some specific forms of weakness may require special approaches: for example, weakness of muscles of swallowing or speech (see p. 65), paralysis of respiratory muscles and diaphragm leading to hypoventilation and hypoxia (see p. 71), or dropped head syndrome.

Dropped head syndrome is a relatively early symptom in some cases of ALS, and relates to a selective weakness of neck extensors. It can lead to difficulty in breathing, and major problems with swallowing (a cause of social embarrassment). The use of a support may be necessary, and a simple soft collar may be adequate; other models that support the head are open at the front to avoid compression of the throat and so allow a little anterior–posterior movement, while preventing lateral movements. When there is more advanced weakness, positioning needs consideration to minimize the effects of gravity, lying the patient in a reclining posture sufficiently far back to prevent any risk of body or head flopping forwards, with support to both sides of the head.

Weakened muscles can rarely be strengthened, but the elasticity of muscle groups, and the range of movement in joints can be sustained, along with the prevention of permanent deformity. While muscle power remains adequate, patients should be encouraged to move the limbs regularly through the day; later the movements will need some assistance, or require passive exercises and gentle stretching carried out by a carer on the advice of a physiotherapist. Lying in bed, for example, weakened leg muscles allow the foot to fall into plantar flexion and this may cause pain in stretched anterior shin muscles and risk stiffness at the ankle joint. Splinting in position, along with regular passive movements, will enhance comfort and prevent deformity.

For everyday activities, the maintenance of independence in the face of progressive weakness will be assisted by an occupational therapist, who will advise on environmental changes: ramps, and alterations to lift the height of chair, bed or toilet seat, or will arrange the installation of rails, a shower chair or commode.

To transfer between bed and chair or wheelchair is a critical part of maintaining quality of life for many weak and dependent individuals. Aids to maintain this ability include bed rails, grips and slippery sheets. Education for patient and carers in techniques for moving to and from a chair is a basic need. An electric wheelchair may need to allow a reclining position for an individual with generalized weakness; a powered hospital-type bed (if necessary with an inflatable mattress) also allows some control of movement that would otherwise be impossible. Sometimes community support groups assist with the provision of such expensive items in the home. If a lifter or hoist is to be sited in the home for very dependent individuals it needs careful selection and trial from among the several types available to ensure that it is safe and comfortable to operate.

Cleaning the perineum after use of the toilet presents difficulties; moistened tissues or cloth towels will be easier for carers to use, and more effective than dry toilet paper.

Wrist splints, and shoulder or arm supports that overcome the effect of gravity can allow better use of weakened distal muscles of the upper limb so that food can be carried to the mouth or a computer keyboard used more effectively. Keyboards and telephones may need modification. Enlarged handles can be more readily grasped, and very light utensils and tools for daily usage, perhaps with the addition of holding devices such as a palmar cuff to assist grip on a spoon or knife, maintain independence.

The patient with major muscle weakness will fatigue easily, and any period of muscular effort will be followed by a time of exhaustion. The patient needs to prioritize activities, and not set ambitious goals for activity.

Terminal phase

In the final stages of a terminal illness, weakness may be too advanced to allow any independent movement, or to maintain respiration (see Assisted ventilation in Chapter 4 of this section, p. 72) or swallowing (see Dysphagia in Chapter 3 of this section, p. 65). To be unable to change position is most uncomfortable, exposing the pressure areas to damage, ulceration and persistent pain, promoting muscle atrophy or spasm and fixing joints so that even assisted movement causes discomfort. The use of air mattresses with a pump that regularly inflates and deflates individual mattress air cells protects the skin; regular passive movements of the limbs and the use of electrically powered beds to allow frequent changes in position will prevent distress. To achieve satisfactory comfort may require additional analgesia and sedation, and a continuous subcutaneous (S/C) infusion over 24 h with small doses of morphine (5–15 mg) and midazolam (5–15 mg) or clonazepam (0.5–2 mg) will often be appreciated by the patient, the attending staff and family.

DISORDERS OF MUSCLE TONE AND CONTRACTION

Muscle dysfunction encompasses a variety of conditions including spasticity, dystonia, rigidity, myoclonus, muscle spasm and posturing.

Spasticity

Spasticity is a velocity-dependent increase in muscle tone with exaggerated tendon reflexes. It follows damage at spinal or supra-spinal levels in the nervous system, commonly seen in cerebral palsy, or caused by traumatic injury to the brain or spinal cord, MS or stroke. Spasticity leads to inappropriate contraction, going on to permanent shortening of muscle bellies, joint contractures and immobility.

The main consequences of spasticity are its effect on mobility and posture. Minor degrees of spasticity may not be apparent at rest, but be observed as marked changes to gait when walking. Persistent spasms cause muscles to become shortened, and contractures occur within them, leading to abnormal mechanical stresses on joints and limbs, and further potentially preventable disability.

Palliation in the supportive phase

The first step in the palliation of spasticity is prevention, avoiding factors that provoke muscle spasm. Spasms can occur spontaneously or as a result of stimulation, such as an alteration in position, being moved, feeling the weight of bedclothes on a limb, coughing or sneezing. Any nociceptive stimulus or abnormal sensory input, for example pain from a pressure ulcer, a full bladder or urinary tract infection, may be a trigger for spasm. Experimentation to reduce those sensory inputs that induce spasm will be important for dexterity, continence and sexual activity, and will assist carers by lessening their burden and the time spent in assisting daily activities. For the patient, success in preventing spasm can lead to improved sleep, reduced pain and avoidance of contractures; effort spent in re-education and rehabilitation will lessen the need to depend on pharmaceutical or surgical measures.

Medications for the relief of spasticity may not be necessary or even desirable. A marked reduction in muscle tone will not always be in the best interests of the patient. If muscles are weak, spasticity can sometimes maintain a degree of stiffness to keep the joints straight and allow weight bearing for transfers from chair to bed, etc. and even help patients walk.

Rehabilitation under the guidance of a multi-disciplinary team will encourage active and passive muscle stretching with the aim to improve mobility, and ensure comfort in posture and during transfer, as well as paying careful attention to bladder and bowel function. Podiatry care, avoidance of tight clothing, and careful use of splints and braces will all contribute.

Pain is a major consequence of muscle spasm and spasticity. Sharp pain can be experienced with acute muscle spasm, and with movement of a body part, but pain also occurs at rest or with lying on a spastic limb. It is often poorly localized, and its mechanisms are not well understood, but is probably best regarded as neuropathic in type, and treated with regular analgesics (from the World Health Organization (WHO) ladder, p. 99) as well as membrane stabilizers (pp. 106–107).

Autonomic pathways may be similarly affected, and spasm of the external bladder sphincter is a common consequence of spinal cord damage, leading to retention of urine (see Urinary retention in Chapter 6 of this section):

Many patients find passive stretching of joints or intermittent standing (in a frame, if need be) helpful in reducing spasms.

Phenol introduced intrathecally to create a chemical rhizotomy can be very effective in relieving spasms and improving opposition in a limb that has no useful function. Clearly this is an intervention that requires both experience and care if complications are to be avoided.

The potential armamentarium includes many medications, of which dantrolene, baclofen and diazepam are most commonly used, starting with low doses and increasing gradually. Many patients cannot achieve a good effect on spasticity without uncomfortable side-effects (notably reduction in consciousness), and randomized-controlled trial evidence for the effectiveness of oral regimens is poor; nevertheless these regimens are commonly used:

- *baclofen 10 and 25 mg tab.*: 5 mg bd, increasing to up to 100 mg in 24 h. Side-effects include drowsiness, increased or painful urination, nausea, confusion and muscle weakness. Sudden withdrawal may precipitate a seizure.
- *dantrolene 25 and 50 mg cap.; 20 mg inj.*: This is often preferred for spasticity of central origin (e.g. from cerebral palsy) starting at 25 mg/day up to 400 mg. Liver toxicity is an occasional but serious idiosyncratic side-effect.
- *diazepam 2 and 5 mg tab.; 5 and 10 mg inj.*: From 5 to 40 mg/day.

Also used are:

- *clonazepam 0.5 mg tab.; 1 mg inj.* 1–6 mg/day.
- *tizanidine* 4–18 mg/day.

All these medications may cause drowsiness.

Tetrahydrocannabinol tab. 2.5–15 mg/day, or cannabis leaf, either smoked or incorporated in cookies, has been claimed to improve spasticity better than placebo, and may be available to, and preferred by, some patients, particularly those still able to walk, even though it is commonly subject to legal restraints.

Failure to respond to oral medications will lead to consideration of more invasive procedures – peripheral nerve blocks (with alcohol or phenol) or 5% phenol injection of motor points where stimulation induces contraction.

While purposeful movement is maintained in some part of even only one hand, it may be possible to direct a powered wheelchair, or manipulate certain electronic devices for entertainment or communication. The usefulness of such equipment will depend often on the level of cognitive function and previous experience and confidence, but when it can be mastered to allow even small amounts of self-directed activity it can be a source of considerable satisfaction.

Botulinum toxin

Injection of botulinum toxin has become a popular treatment in some medical facilities for certain forms of muscle spasm and spasticity. It induces weakness in striated muscles by inhibiting transmission at the neuromuscular junction. It also inhibits release of acetylcholine in autonomic neurones, and so affects overactive smooth muscles (e.g. in achalasia) and reduces the activity of glands. The terminal axon of the neurone sprouts new motor endplates; therefore, the effects of the toxin wane with time and reinnervation generally occurs within 3–4 months. Unintended weakness of muscles that are uninvolved may occur if they are inadvertently injected or affected by diffusion from the injection site.

Botulinum toxin, available as 100 or 500 U pack, has to be injected into affected muscles or glands. Doses are tailored to individual patients, guided by the mass of muscle being injected. Susceptibility to the toxin varies. Each muscle must be injected separately. Injection into salivary glands will reduce the pharyngeal accumulation of secretions and drooling in persons who can no longer swallow effectively. Local injection is a very effective treatment for local hyperhidrosis, such as commonly affects a spastic clenched hand.

Overactive muscles are located by identifying hypertrophy, tenderness and abnormal activity, sometimes with the assistance of electromyography. Patients usually experience initial relief and then gradually deteriorate to a point where a further injection is required, the interval and the dose varying widely.

Botulinum toxin is also used for reducing painful bladder spasms by being introduced per urethra into the bladder cavity.

Due to expense, in most countries medical insurance or government funding for the use of botulinum toxin is restricted to a small set of indications (such as blepharospasm, hemifacial spasm and torticollis). Injections for several persons may be arranged on the same day to make best use of one batch, because of its short half-life. In MS it does not consistently improve functional outcomes, and the high cost may not justify its use.

Other interventions undertaken to improve comfort included tenotomy, tendon lengthening and transfer procedures and correction of deformities. Whether such interventions are appropriate in any particular case will depend on the assessment of discomfort being experienced, the prognosis and patient and family expectations. Where painful spasms persist in spite of other treatments, microsurgical techniques at the dorsal root entry area have been tried, with variable results.

Intrathecal baclofen

Baclofen is lipophilic and crosses the blood–brain barrier poorly, and therefore is ideal for intrathecally administration in a daily dose of 100–300 μg, the much reduced dose diminishing side-effects. Continuous intrathecal administration of baclofen via an implanted pump aims to provide long-term beneficial effect on disabling spasticity, but the measure lacks the support of rigorously derived evidence. The procedure does not reduce voluntary motor function. The implanted pump is expensive and requires careful supervision and monitoring to avoid overdosage. Reported infection rates vary from 0% to 18% and prophylactic antibiotics may be suggested to cover the period following pump placement.

Palliation in the terminal phase

Established muscle contractures are a common accompaniment of advanced neurological deterioration in a number of diseases in which mobility and cognition are both impaired. Joints fixed by muscle contractures make many movements painful and difficult, and the avoidance of pressure ulcers requires diligent nursing. Nutrition will commonly be impaired when there is no capacity to self-feed, and positioning for swallowing becomes difficult.

A crumpled, wasted immobile body can be a source of persistent pain. Continuous S/C administration of analgesic and sedation (see Medications for pain management in Chapter 7 of this section, p. 98) may be an appropriate means to ensure comfort at this time.

Rigidity is a velocity-independent resistance to stretch in skeletal muscle, typical of Parkinson's disease and its associated syndromes (see chapter Parkinson's Disease and Related Disorders of Section III, p. 142).

Dystonia

Dystonia is sustained involuntary contraction of muscle and may be focal, segmental, multifocal or generalized producing abnormal posture with frequent twisting and turning. It may affect the extremities with over-extension or over-flexion of the hand, or inversion of the foot, and can cause twisting, lateral bending and torsion of the spine. It has many underlying causes, some primary and with a genetic basis, others associated with Parkinson's diseases or other neurological degenerative conditions, still others secondary to brain damage from trauma, infection or malignancy. Neuroleptic drugs (phenothiazines, haloperidol) and dopamine antagonists should be excluded as a cause.

In the management of dystonia, anticholinergic drugs, clonazepam or carbamazepine may have some limited benefit:

- *benzhexol 2 mg, 5 mg tab.* up to 5 mg once daily or bd or
- *benztropine 2 mg tab.; 2 mg/ml inj.* 2 mg once daily or bd (but side-effects limit use in older persons);
- *clonazepam 0.5, 2 mg tab.* 1–4 mg/24 h;
- *carbamazepine 100, 200, 400 mg tab.; 20 mg/ml susp.* 200–1200 mg/24 h.

Otherwise drug treatment is very similar to what is recommended for spasticity, and is subject to the same limitations of unsatisfactory response or unwelcome side-effects in many instances. Unlike spasticity, dystonia does not respond to intrathecal administration of baclofen.

Botulinum toxin may be selectively injected into dystonic limbs, especially when the fist becomes forcibly clenched and functionally useless.

Focal and segmental dystonia includes blepharospasm, cervical dystonia (spasmodic torticollis) and spasmodic dysphonia. These can be treated by injection of botulinum toxin into the affected muscles, repeated every 3 months.

Muscle cramps

Muscle cramps are a common problem in everyday life, and are usually not associated with any underlying serious disorder. They may be a feature of disorders of sodium and calcium, and occasionally will occur in neurological conditions where there is denervation or corticospinal spasticity:

- *quinine 300 mg* in a single evening dose for the common night time cramps that affect the elderly has been popular and effective. However, its use is associated with a 1–3% incidence of haematological abnormalities, particularly thrombocytopenia and this has led to its discontinuation in some countries.
- *baclofen 10 mg and 25 mg tab*. 5–10 mg bd or tds or
- *orphenadrine 100 mg tab*. 100 mg bd or tds may be more effective for resistant cramps.

SEIZURES

Seizures are dramatic events. While health professionals tend to regard seizure disorders as episodic, people affected by them know that the ever-present threat of a seizure with loss of awareness, loss of control and loss of dignity, along with the consequent restrictions on their life, are persistent.

The classification of epilepsy and of seizure type is complex and dynamic. Generalized seizures affect consciousness and may be associated with loss of posture and shaking of all four limbs ('generalized tonic–clonic') or be confined to brief periods of loss of awareness ('absences'). Partial seizures affect one part of the brain and its function (e.g. speech, or a single limb movement). Sometimes a seizure may begin as a partial seizure but then spread to become generalized.

Treatment of people with life-long generalized seizures has a high rate of success; treatment for partial seizures arising in the context of a neurological condition is much less successful. In addition, metabolic changes or drug treatment in the later stages of care can precipitate seizures. Clinicians should maintain a heightened index of suspicion that seizures might occur in cerebral tumour, following trauma or in conditions such as liver failure, uraemia, hypoglycaemia, hyperthyroid or hypoparathyroid states, all of which may lower the threshold at which a seizure occurs. The administration or withdrawal of drugs (e.g. alcohol, barbiturates) also may increase the risk of seizure. Repeated use of meperidine (pethidine) in chronic pain, can lead to an accumulation of nor-meperidine and induction of seizures.

Status epilepticus may be generalized (convulsive status) or partial. It is a serious situation in which seizure follows seizure without recovery in between. This has the potential to increase damage to the brain, and convulsive status can be life threatening. Some forms of partial status are difficult to recognize when presenting as episodic confusion or as a behavioural change, abrupt in onset and termination and varying in duration. An electroencephalogram (EEG) recorded during an episode can be helpful and intravenous (I-V) benzodiazepines usually bring the episode to an end.

The manifestations of seizures may be predominantly motor, sensory or psychological, and be so subtle and complex as to require considerable neurological expertise for their elucidation.

Palliation of seizures in the supportive phase
Pre-existing epilepsy

Some patients requiring palliative care for a neurological condition will also have experienced seizures throughout their life. The diagnosis will be clear; treatment already in place should continue while oral medication remains practicable. A small proportion will have seizures that are truly refractory; for these persons the advice of their neurologist should be sought as he/she may already have encountered the problem and be able to advise the best approach to treatment.

Deterioration in the control of previously well-controlled seizures should alert the clinician to the possibility of infection, metabolic disturbance and a new drug treatment (or drug withdrawal). While seeking to correct any metabolic or pharmacological cause, the dose of medication should be increased, unless already at the maximum tolerated dose, when it would be wise to solicit the advice of the supervising neurologist before adding or replacing medication.

Seizures arising as part of the neurological condition

Primary or secondary brain tumours and stroke are particularly likely to give rise to seizures, usually partial, arising in the region of damage to the brain, but may become secondarily generalized. Partial seizures may be succeeded by a prolonged period of worsened focal neurological features (e.g. Todd's paresis).

Not every person with a progressive cerebral tumour will suffer seizures and prophylactic anti-epileptic drugs are not universally recommended. Rather is it usual to warn attendants of the risk, give simple instruction in first-aid measures, and to begin regular anti-epileptic therapy only if a first seizure has occurred.

The onset of seizures in the later stages of a neurological condition deserves investigation because upsets such as a low calcium level or hypoxia lessen the success of drug therapy.

Management of seizures

Seizures are frightening to the individual and to onlookers and carers. They often further impair the quality of life. Sympathetic explanation and advice should be given throughout the stages of diagnosis and treatment. Neurological advice should be sought wherever there is difficulty in establishing a cause or controlling seizures.

Treatment begins with steps to reduce harm and protect the airway, moving the patient away from sources of danger and employing the recovery position as soon as possible. Individual seizures are usually self-limiting and no other treatment is required. If a seizure persists longer than 15 min an I-V benzodiazepine should be given, for example:

- *diazepam 10 mg inj.* 10 mg I-V,
- *clonazepam 1 mg inj.* 1 mg I-V.

Failure to respond after a further dose 15 min later suggests that the procedure for status epilepticus should be followed (v.i.). Rectal administration is a measure some carers can learn to use where prolonged seizures occur frequently:

- *diazepam 10 mg, susp. or inj.* 10 mg delivered via a plastic tube.

Status epilepticus

When generalized seizure follows seizure without recovery in between, there is potential for increased brain damage and even a threat to life. The airway should be secured and I-V treatment should be given immediately the situation is recognized, with a benzodiazepine or phenytoin:

- *clonazepam 1 mg inj.* 1–2 mg I-V, and repeat after 15 minutes if necessary;
- *phenytoin 100, 250 mg inj.* 20 mg/kg given at a rate of 50 mg/min.

Neurological and critical care advice and support should be sought to ensure that ventilation is maintained, unless it has already been decided that further treatment would not be appropriate. However, the distress caused to family and friends by continuing seizures is considerable.

Consideration always should be given to trying to arrest the seizures, using I-V barbiturates (thiopentone) or propofol if the previously mentioned drugs have been ineffective. The risk of suppressing respiration should be carefully explained to the family and carers.

I-V benzodiazepines usually abort partial status, but the difficulties in diagnosing and managing this group of seizures suggests the need for further neurological advice if the seizures continue.

Prophylactic treatment
- *valproate 100, 200, 500 mg tab.; 200 mg/ml susp.* (600–2000 mg/day) is usually preferred for generalized seizures. Blood levels are not useful or necessary. Either valproate or carbamazepine are recommended for partial seizures.
- *carbamazepine 100, 200, 400 mg tab.; 20 mg/ml susp.* Start at a dose of 100 mg bd, and increase gradually to the dose necessary to gain control or produce side-effects (usually 600–1200 mg/day), checking blood levels.
- *phenobarbitone 200 mg/1 ml amp.* 200–300 mg is an alternative for I-V or S/C administration.
- *phenytoin 30, 100 mg cap.; 50 mg tab.; 50 mg/ml inj.* 200–500 mg daily.

Second line oral maintenance treatments include lamotrigine, topiramate, clobazam and phenobarbitone.

There are many important pharmacological interactions between anti-epileptic drugs and medications used in palliative care. Phenytoin and carbamazepine induce liver enzymes and interfere with the metabolism of both warfarin (used for venous thrombosis) and corticosteroids (cerebral tumour). The action of phenytoin itself is affected by cimetidine and omeprazole (oesophageal reflux not uncommon with weight gain and recumbent posture), imipramine (used for neuropathic pain) and ketoconazole (resistant oral and oesophageal moniliasis).

Palliation of seizures in the terminal phase
In view of the distress caused to the individual and to carers, family and friends every effort should be made to keep seizures under control. A reduction in consciousness, or direct patient refusal may lead to an inability to administer oral medication. Phenytoin and, in some countries, valproate can be administered by I-V route, but the most convenient medications are

those available for regular administration by the S/C route:

- *clonazepam 0.5, 2 mg tab.; 1 mg/ml inj.* 1–2 mg daily or bd by intermittent injection or as a continuous S/C infusion (2–4 mg/ 24 h);
- *phenobarbitone 200 mg/ml* 200–300 mg daily or bd by S/C bolus injection may also assist, dose and frequency of administration being increased as necessary to achieve control. Status epilepticus occurring at this stage should be treated as above.

INVOLUNTARY MOVEMENTS

Myoclonus

Myoclonus is an irregular, rapid multifocal contraction of part or all of a muscle, occurring either spontaneously or in response to a stimulus or voluntary movement. It can be a manifestation of epilepsy or occur in a number of other conditions, including degenerative diseases, some genetic conditions and as a result of local ischaemia, a metabolic upset or drug administration. It may cause relatively little distress, or be associated with hyperalgesia and allodynia. Periodic twitching of the lower limb flexor muscles during sleep is not uncommon in persons unaffected by any major disease, and may cause multiple awakenings during the night, or leave the patient unaware (see Restless legs in Chapter 2 of this section, p. 60).

Myoclonus is a relatively common adverse effect of opioid administration, variably dose dependent, and is managed by a reduction in dose, a change in the opioid, or a change in the route of administration, or both:

- *valproate and clonazepam* (within the dose range used for epilepsy) are useful for reducing the frequency and extent of contractions, if the need for pain control with opioids requires continuation of high doses causing myoclonus;
- *clonazepam 1 mg/ml* can be administered by S/C bolus or infusion.

Tremor

Tremor is a rhythmic, mechanical oscillation of at least one body region, occurring in association with disease affecting the basal ganglia, brainstem, cerebellum or peripheral nervous system. It can range from imperceptible physiological movements to a severe shaking causing great handicap.

Common tremor presentations include:

- resting tremor, a manifestation of Parkinson's disease in younger patients (see p. 143);

- intention tremor – an indication of cerebellar involvement and is commonly seen in MS (see p. 137);
- essential tremor;
- metabolic tremor (e.g. 'liver flap') and the fine tremor of thyrotoxicosis. These are outside the range of this discussion.

Resting tremor may be mild, or quite disabling and a major embarrassment. Where it is the major manifestation of the disease in younger patients, anticholinergic drugs will reduce the symptom:

- *benzhexol 2, 5 mg tab.* up to 5 mg once daily or bd or
- *benztropine 2 mg tab.; 2 mg/ml inj.* 2 mg once daily or bd, but side-effects limit use in older persons.

Dopamine agonists by mouth:

- *bromocriptine 2.5 mg tab.; 5, 10 mg cap.* up to 15 mg bd;
- *pergolide 50, 200 µg, 1 mg.* up to 1 mg bd are best reserved for younger patients, who withstand the side-effects better (nausea, hypotension, dreams and hallucinations and sleepiness). Severe nausea will often be relieved by domperidone 10 mg.

   Intention tremor and ataxia occur with cerebellar involvement with associated clumsiness and an increased risk of falls. Management of intention tremor is mostly unsatisfactory. In very mild cases the use of weights in a sleeve or a heavy wristband is helpful:

- *clonazepam* is probably the most helpful drug (0.5–6 mg/24 h); alternatives are baclofen 10–25 mg orally, three times daily or
- *carbamazepine* 100 mg orally, twice daily, slowly increasing until symptoms resolve or to 300 mg twice daily.

Cannabis compounds are also popular in some quarters (p. 52).

   Essential tremor may be familial or occur late in life. It is often bilateral, affecting hands and forearms, or the head. As an isolated disorder it should be treated only when it impairs ability to perform activities. Relaxation therapy may assist, or a single standard drink of alcohol:

- *propranolol 10, 40 mg tab.* 10 mg orally, twice daily, increasing to 240 mg daily or
- *primidone 250 mg tab.* 62.5 mg orally, at night, up to 125–250 mg twice daily, will have a helpful effect;

- *topiramate 50, 100, 200 mg tab.; 15, 25, 50 mg sprinkle cap.* 25–50 mg twice daily is also effective.

Restless legs

'Restless legs' is the name commonly given to a syndrome of unpleasant limb sensations precipitated by rest and relieved by activity. Symptoms are worse at night and may cause insomnia. The discomfort is often described as a crawling, tingling, burning or aching sensation rather than a pain. Voluntary activity such as stretching the legs or pacing the floor gives relief, and massage to the legs or a hot bath may assist.

The syndrome occurs in members of the general population who have no underlying recognized cause, but is also more common in peripheral neuropathy, lumbosacral radiculopathies, myelopathies and Parkinson's disease. Useful medications taken before going to bed include benzodiazepines:

- *clonazepam 0.5 – 2 mg;*
- *temazepam 10, 20 mg tab.; 10, 20 mg cap.* 7.5–30 mg; or
- *carbidopa–levodopa (25 mg carbidopa + 100, 250 mg levodopa)* 1 tab.;
- *pergolide 50, 200 μg, 1 mg* a dopamine agonist, increasing from a dose of 50 μg.

The use of many other medications is described in the literature; recent reports claim benefit for ropinirole. The multiple agents suggested may indicate that no single agent is uniformly effective.

A reduction in caffeine and alcohol intake and cessation of smoking is also advised.

DRUG-INDUCED MOVEMENT DISORDERS

Dopamine antagonists (e.g. haloperidol, prochlorperazine and metoclopramide) may cause parkinsonism, acute dystonia, tardive dyskinesia, neuroleptic malignant syndrome, akathisia and restlessness. Acute forms of these disorders respond to anticholinergics or cessation of the causative drugs; chronic forms respond poorly. Presentation can range from very subtle symptoms of distress or restlessness through to florid and bizarre movements and behaviour. A medication effect should be suspected and the drug dose reduced or alternative medications introduced. If treating an acute psychotic reaction, for example, prefer clozapine, which carries a much reduced risk of movement disorder.

Relief of the symptoms may be effected with:

- *benztropine 2 mg tab.; 2 mg/ml inj.* 1–2 mg orally, intramuscular (I-M) or I-V;
- *benzhexol 2, 5 mg tab.* 2 mg orally or
- *biperiden 2 mg tab.* 1 mg orally.

Serotonin syndrome

Neuromuscular hyperactivity is one feature of serotonin syndrome in which there is excessive accumulation of serotonin in the nervous system following the administration of drugs that may be used for palliation of other discomforts. They either promote serotonin release (e.g. amphetamines, monoamine oxidase inhibitors), inhibit its re-uptake (SSRI antidepressants, some opioids) or stimulate its receptors (bromocriptine, buspirone).

Agitation, delirium or seizures and autonomic dysfunction also characterize the syndrome, and serious complications such as hyperthermia, renal failure and disseminated intravascular coagulation are possible. I-V fluids and assisted ventilation may be necessary, cyproheptadine and chlorpromazine are serotonin receptor antagonists and help abort the condition.

Hemifacial spasm

This condition is due most often to neurovascular compression of the facial nerve in the posterior fossa. If treatment is sought because of social disability, surgical decompression of the facial nerve may be done for younger patients, alternatively regular injections of botulinum toxin into the affected muscles are likely to be effective.

Tardive dyskinesia

Patients on long-term typical antipsychotic medication may develop tardive dyskinesia, a complex syndrome of involuntary hyperkinetic movements, usually large in amplitude, irregular and worsened with distraction. It most frequently affects the mouth, lips, tongue and jaws, with smacking, tongue writhing, sucking or chewing movements and tic-like movements of the lips, eyes and facial muscles. The limbs and trunk can be affected with choreoathetoid movements. The abnormal movements disappear in sleep. They interfere with breathing, speaking and eating. Women, older persons, those with past brain injury and those with mood disorders are at increased risk.

Due to the lack of suitable management for established tardive dyskinesia, prevention is clearly preferred. Antipsychotic drugs should only be used in the lowest effective dose and only in those patients where there is a strong clinical indication.

The course of tardive dyskinesia is variable. There is a substantial group of patients in whom it is irreversible. It is, therefore, important to regularly monitor patients on antipsychotic drugs for early signs of tardive dyskinesia.

SYNCOPE AND FALLS

Impaired mental status, special toileting needs, impaired mobility and the use of medications that affect the central nervous system all contribute to a high risk of falling in neurological disease. Poor vision and an orthostatic fall in blood pressure (BP) (often exaggerated by drug therapy), plus environmental factors such as poor lighting, slippery floor coverings and unsafe footwear further increase that risk. Falls are particularly prevalent in persons with Parkinson's disease, syncope due to cardiovascular pathologies (transient ischaemic attack (TIAs), bradyarrhythmias or post-cerebro-vascular accident (CVA), Alzheimer's disease or polyneuropathy). They are also seen in extrapyramidal syndromes such as progressive supra-nuclear palsy (PSP) and multi-system atrophy (MSA) (Shy–Drager) and the autonomic neuropathies.

Measures to reduce any orthostatic fall in BP in MSA include anti-G-suits, compressive stockings, increased salt intake, elevating the head of the bed and fludrocortisone, and can improve activity and independence. Falls are common with the decrease in muscle strength and joint flexibility seen in ALS, MS and muscular dystrophy.

More than one-half of persons with neurological disease who fall have a disturbance of gait; others have epileptic seizures, episodes of syncope or have suffered a stroke. The stiffness of movement found in Parkinson's disease predisposes patients to fall in a backward or medial–lateral direction; poorly directed arm movements and freezing of gait also contribute to falls.

Repeated falls are a burden not only for the patient, but also for the caregivers and the health system. Falls and instability threaten safety and independence and are major reasons for nursing home admission.

A simple test for the risk of falling is to do no more than ask a person to get up from bed and walk to a wheelchair, allowing assessment of strength, gait and balance. A more comprehensive assessment by a physiotherapist should guide any programme of prevention.

To decrease falls, it is necessary to identify and correct the major determinant factors and seek to remove potential hazards. Particularly important will be a review of medications. For example, those patients with

Parkinson's disease who responded well to levodopa have been shown to be more likely to fall. In the terminal stage of an illness, many prescribed medications may be doing more harm than good, and it is not uncommon to note some improvement following the cessation of medications that have been used for months and years.

A careful assessment of the environment should be undertaken to ensure the appropriate placement and height of furniture, grab rails and bars. The use of treaded slipper socks may be useful. Exercise has been shown to have a beneficial effect in reducing falls, but not in adults who have significant cognitive impairment.

Bulbar symptoms

IMPAIRED SPEECH

Speech is a complex motor function involving respiratory effort, vocal cord movement, and activity of the lips, tongue, pharynx and palate. There are many possible ways in which it may be inhibited, leading to a frustrating inability to utter clear words, the sounds being slurred, weak or aspirate, and quickly exhausting the patient.

The contribution of speech therapy/pathology

Speech therapy (sometimes described as speech pathology) is an important potential palliative intervention, offering a comprehensive assessment and suggestions for improving patient capacity and staff understanding. Tests of hearing and vision, assessment of receptive abilities, motor functions, cognitive and emotional capacity may all be important.

There are many devices that augment communication, using voice amplification, writing, drawings, picture boards and whiteboards. Electronic devices provide synthetic speech for words entered into a word processor or scan eye movements as focus switches from one word or letter to another. But even the most sophisticated machines are far slower than normal speech and require both patience and close attention on the part of both parties to the communication. For this reason, the most helpful persons are those who engage with the patient frequently, and who learn individual idiosyncrasies as the struggle to appreciate and make wants known proceeds. They may be family members or trained volunteers. Particularly in the terminal phase, the presence of just a few persons whom the patient has learnt to trust and rely on will be most appreciated.

DYSPHAGIA

The process of swallowing is a highly integrated sequence involving many muscles, both voluntary and involuntary. Difficulty in transferring a bolus of food from the mouth to the stomach (dysphagia) may be of obstructive or neurogenic origin. Problems in the control of other muscles contribute when they result, for example, in inability to hold the head up, denying the useful effect of gravity.

Dysphagia can lead to excessive drooling, to choking and regurgitation, to a sense of food sticking in the pharynx or oesophagus, to malnutrition, weight loss and a significant risk of aspiration pneumonia.

Among many contributions to swallowing difficulty are dryness of the mouth, and medications such as benzodiazepines or dopamine antagonists.

Neurological causes include stroke, brain injury, Parkinson's disease, dementia, cerebral neoplasms, Huntington's disease, Wilson's disease, torticollis, motor neurone disease (MND), multiple sclerosis (MS), polyneuritis, myasthenia, muscular dystrophy and poliomyelitis.

It is common to distinguish bulbar palsy, in which lower motor neurones below the level of the Vth nerve nucleus in the mid-pons medulla are affected, from pseudobulbar palsy, due to bilateral cortico-bulbar lesions. In pseudobulbar palsy there is incoordination out of proportion to the weakness observed, and the ingestion of fluids causes more difficulty than solids.

Lesions affecting predominantly the oropharynx lead to drooling, impaired chewing, nasal regurgitation, coughing, choking and food sticking in the throat. There are persistent attempts to clear the throat, and the voice sounds 'wet'.

When the difficulty is mainly in the oesophagus there is a sensation of food sticking in chest, with regurgitation, heartburn and chest discomfort.

In either case, potential complications include dehydration, malnutrition, laryngo-spasm, broncho-spasm and aspiration pneumonia.

Dysphagia problems are prominent in particular neurological conditions, including:

- Myasthenia gravis, in which tongue weakness makes it difficult to gather into a firm bolus foods placed in the mouth.
- Amyotrophic lateral sclerosis (ALS)/MND, where there is weak chewing, nasal regurgitation, a poor gag reflex and incomplete vocal cord adduction leading to aspiration.
- Huntington's disease, in which choreiform movements compromise feeding and swallowing. It is hard to place food in the mouth, a vigorous tongue may push it out, chewing is laboured, solids are handled better than liquids. Unpredictable gulping of air opens the glottis and predisposes to aspiration.
- Parkinson's disease in which medication administration should be timed to give best control of movements at meal times.

Principles of management of dysphagia in neurological diseases include:

- Establish optimal possible communication with the patient to achieve mutual understanding of the plan of treatment, and patiently reinforce each step.
- Carefully position the trunk, sitting up, and find the best position of the head (tilting or turning).
- Avoid distractions, so that the patient concentrates on swallowing.
- Prepare the mouth by suction of thick mucus, moistening with water.
- Offer a safe and enticing diet to stimulate chewing and swallowing. Tests of swallowing can safely be made with spoons of crushed ice; thickened fluids and fine minces are often better managed than watery fluids. Food should be offered in small amounts, with encouragement of thorough chewing and slow eating, washing each mouthful down with fluid, and making a double swallow, all of which assist effective swallowing.

Speech therapists work to improve swallowing by offering useful advice about food presentation and consistency, the position of the trunk and head during swallowing attempts, and exercises to improve chewing and the delivery of food through the pharynx to the oesophagus.

The use of simple aids – a plastic squeeze bottle, a non-slip disc for holding a cup on a tray, a cup with a nose cut-out, or a high-rimmed dish to help load a spoon may all assist confidence. Other available devices assist a weak hand to hold a spoon or support the arms to lift food to the mouth.

When nutrition is clearly compromised, a naso-gastric tube may be suggested. But this blocks the nose, forces mouth breathing and a dry mouth, and interferes with the sensations needed for swallowing. Depending on the prognosis and the wishes of patient and family, a per-endoscopic gastrostomy (PEG) may be a better option. If the patient has a dread of eating because of the discomfort that follows attempts to swallow, a gastrostomy should be considered.

The aim of a feeding regimen will often be to provide 1.0–1.2 kcal/kg and 0.8–1.0 g/kg of protein in 1.0–2.5 l every 24 h. In advanced disease, such a programme of feeding may be quite unrealistic, or inappropriate. If the emphasis is on comfort rather than prolongation of survival, restriction of intake to the foods and the quantities that can easily be handled by the patient is a desirable approach.

If dehydration becomes severe (as in hot weather) subcutaneous (S/C) fluids (1 l of normal saline over 24 h) may be sufficient to maintain comfort.

FEAR OF CHOKING

In situations where there is progressive impairment of respiratory effort and voluntary swallowing, patients and families may express fears of 'choking to death' in the last throes of ALS or muscular dystrophy. Such fear is largely unfounded, and if accumulation of pharyngeal secretions seems to threaten major distress, the use of injections of opioid, together with an anxiolytic such as midazolam and an anticholinergic (hyoscine) will restore comfort:

- *morphine 5–10 mg + midazolam 2.5–5 mg + hyoscine hydrobromide 0.4 mg.*

In the UK, a 'Breathing Space Kit' was developed by the Motor Neurone Association to make these medications available for carers to store at home and have confidence to use them in times of crisis.

DROOLING

The salivary glands in a healthy individual secrete up to 1.5 l of saliva per day; 90% from the parotid and submandibular glands. Saliva facilitates swallowing, keeps the mouth moist, acts as a solvent for molecules that stimulate the taste buds and keeps the mouth and teeth clean, providing some protection against dental caries.

Drooling is not due to increased production of saliva, but results from a poor oral (lip) seal and poor tongue coordination, often accompanied by impaired swallowing that results in saliva pooling in the oropharynx. There is a consequent risk of overflow and aspiration.

Children with cerebral palsy often experience the discomfort of drooling, and intensive efforts can be made to retrain them in more effective oral skills, perhaps with the assistance of a palatal training appliance. Surgical measures may be undertaken to reduce saliva flow, and for these younger patients careful monitoring should be undertaken to prevent problems that may stem from a lack of saliva (such as the development of dental caries).

In adult patients facing a progressive decline, education efforts are less likely to be rewarding, and drooling will be more often managed by anticholinergic drugs to block the autonomic muscarinic receptors. Anticholinergic medications often have side-effects, however, and may not be tolerated by many patients:

- *benztropine 2 mg tab.; 2 mg/ml inj.* 1–2 mg orally, intramuscular (I-M) or intravenous (I-V);

- *glycopyrrolate 0.2 mg/ml*, 1–2 ml S/C;
- *benzhexol 2, 5 mg tab.* 2 mg orally.

All are used for this purpose, but there is no evidence that one drug is preferable.

Botulinum A toxin injection of the salivary glands is a more recently available option. A solution is injected into the salivary gland, and care must be taken to prevent diffusion out from the site of administration. In treatment of hemifacial spasms, blepharospasms and torticollis, diffusion of the fluid has produced unwelcome facial muscle weaknesses and dysphagia.

4

Respiratory symptoms

In neurology, the most common respiratory problem is neuromuscular disease leading to hypoventilation. Respiratory muscles still functioning are called upon to work much harder, leading to muscle pains, anxiety, exhaustion and weight loss. Cough becomes weak and ineffective, secretions accumulate and are difficult to expel, hypoxia and hypercapnoea follow hypoventilation. Hypoventilation is associated with multiple discomforts, including dyspnoea, sleeplessness, daytime fatigue and sleepiness, morning headache, difficulty in phonation and the risk of aspiration pneumonia.

Unlike those who suffer from cardiac or respiratory disease, who experience major respiratory distress, a failing respiration may occur very quietly in neuromuscular disease, with no apparent resultant difficulty in breathing. If this is not recognized, persons suffering from myasthenia gravis or polyneuropathy may develop severe problems before observers realize they are not breathing effectively.

DYSPNOEA

Respiration is a finely balanced automatic process, controlled by multiple receptors sensing posture, lung and airway stretch, blood gases, muscle movement, even odours and airflow. Various kinds of imbalance are possible, and may coexist, upsetting the automatic adjustment of respiratory effort, and causing a feeling that respiratory muscles must work harder to maintain comfort.

Dyspnoea, an uncomfortable awareness of breathing, is a subjective discomfort, and its relationship with objective measures of respiratory function is complicated by the many other factors of circumstance and emotion. It will occur when there is a need for increased respiratory effort (as in lung disease) or an increased ventilatory requirement (as in hypoxaemia, anaemia or metabolic acidosis). In neurological conditions it will be due more often to a decrease in respiratory muscle strength or an alteration of breathing awareness. An anxiety panic attack may cause hyperventilation and induce a sensation of dyspnoea in persons with normal respiratory effort. Conversely, a fan blowing air gently into the face may bring relief to an individual struggling for breath from advanced lung disease.

Assessment of dyspnoea therefore needs a broad approach, taking into account such physical components as vital capacity, lung compliance, alveolar gas exchange, airway obstruction, respiratory muscles and central nervous control; but also considering the emotional, social, environmental and cultural aspects that influence how discomforts are experienced and interpreted.

Treatment will be directed at relief of any remediable cause:

- reassurance or benzodiazepines to counter anxiety,
- re-positioning to a more upright posture,
- bronchodilatators for constricted airways,
- removal of pleural fluid, etc.

Opioid medications (e.g. oral morphine in small doses) will usually have a calming effect and will take away the panic feeling and distress of fighting for breath:

- *morphine 2 mg/ml susp.* 2–10 mg, 2–6 hourly as needed.

When dyspnoea is continual, both opioids and benzodiazepines will provide some relief, either by intermittent oral or subcutaneous (S/C) administration or by continuous infusion:

- *morphine 10–30 mg + midazolam 5–10 mg* over 24 h.

Fear of respiratory depression through the administration of such small doses is unfounded, and both comfort and function are usually enhanced by this approach.

Oxygen may be no more than a useful placebo unless an improvement in hypoxia can be demonstrated, and there is a risk of its causing respiratory depression when there has been longstanding carbon dioxide (CO_2) retention.

HYPOVENTILATION

Alveolar hypoventilation associated with neuromuscular disease can occur acutely, with progressive weakness of respiratory muscles causing a rapid reduction in vital capacity followed by respiratory failure with hypoxaemia and hypercarbia. Symptoms will include dyspnoea, tachypnoea and tachycardia.

More commonly the onset is insidious and chronic, impairment of the respiratory muscles decreasing the ability to clear secretions, and even altering the function of the respiratory centres. Symptoms include orthopnoea, fatigue, disturbed sleep and hypersomnolence. Treatment will address the underlying clinical cause. For stable diseases (old polio, quadriplegia or kyposcoliosis) mechanical support of ventilation can reverse symptoms. For chronic and progressive disease such as muscular dystrophy and amyotrophic lateral sclerosis, mechanical support provides only symptomatic relief and is usually associated with further deterioration and reliance on complete ventilation for survival.

Nocturnal hypoventilation

Nocturnal respiratory failure (hypoventilation) may occur despite normal daytime respiratory function. The normal physiological reduction of muscle tone during sleep may be life threatening in a patient with impaired muscle strength. Evaluation by a sleep study may be useful in a patient with neuromuscular disease in whom there are nocturnal symptoms such as air hunger, intermittent snoring, orthopnoea, cyanosis, restlessness and insomnia. Daytime symptoms may include morning drowsiness, headaches and excessive daytime sleepiness.

If a persistent nocturnal fall in oxygen concentration is demonstrated, medication with nortriptyline or protriptyline and nocturnal oxygen may assist, but many individuals will require non-invasive ventilation such as continuous positive airway pressure, bilevel positive airway pressure (BiPAP), intermittent positive pressure ventilation or, rarely, tracheostomy.

ASSISTED VENTILATION

The need to assist ventilation in persons with neurodegenerative diseases such as post-polio syndrome, amyotrophic lateral sclerosis, myasthenia gravis, myotonic dystrophy and muscular dystrophy will be indicated by the onset of orthopnoea (the patient requiring to be propped up to breathe without dyspnoea) or a blood oxygen less than 65 mm. Nocturnal hypoventilation may be demonstrated by a sleep study and indicate the value of ventilation assistance before daytime hypoxia is obvious.

Non-invasive positive pressure ventilation (NIPPV) via a nasal or nasofacial mask relieves many of the symptoms of hypoventilation, and modern equipment (such as BiPAP) makes NIPPV eminently suitable for home use.

The availability of ventilation and the frequency with which it is offered to patients suffering from hypoventilation has varied from country to country. It is likely to become more widely implemented since it has been shown to increase survival considerably in diseases such as amyotrophic lateral sclerosis (ALS).

NIPPV requires a close fit of the mask to the face to ensure that a small level of positive air pressure will adequately inflate the lungs, and some individuals find this uncomfortable; others, recognizing the progressive nature of their disease and unwilling to extend its discomfort, refuse this assistance. Patients who have bulbar symptoms that prevent adequate cough and expulsion of secretions from the upper airways may be at risk of aspiration, and some do not tolerate non-invasive ventilation, finding that it does not fully remove intermittent sensations of dyspnoea.

Ventilation via a tracheostomy requires 24 h availability of persons trained to watch over the system and the airway, and perform suction when necessary, and therefore, while it can be managed in the home, it is usually limited to patients accommodated in hospital.

Ventilator issues associated with tracheostomy

There are five levels of decision-making involved in the more intrusive ventilation assistance via a tracheostomy:

1. Whether to insert a nasal or oral endotracheal tube either for suction of sticky retained secretions or to allow a temporary assistance with assisted pressure ventilation (perhaps at the time of a chest infection).
2. Whether to re-introduce a nasal or oral endotracheal tube on a similar subsequent occasion. The removal of such a tube will be necessary after a time. It is not a measure that can be done repeatedly.
3. Whether a tracheostomy should be performed, in the event of recurrent or more difficult dyspnoea. Sometimes the tracheostomy is valuable without positive pressure ventilation through reducing dead space and allowing better suction (which families can manage at home after training).
4. Whether assisted ventilation should be introduced via the tracheostomy. For many individuals with ALS or muscular dystrophy invasive ventilation via a tracheostomy can maintain life for a number of years. But care for such support is complex, and if undertaken at home causes significant strain and stress on carers. In some countries it will be the usual final pathway of management, but in both Australia and UK it is performed far less often.
5. Whether this assistance should be withdrawn. An indefinite prolongation of life through this assistance may come to be regarded as onerous, uncomfortable and undesirable. As removal of the

positive pressure support will often lead to death within a short time, many physicians may feel they cannot do this, and in some countries it will be illegal, even when the patient indicates a clear directive.

At each level, there should be careful anticipatory discussion to prepare patient and family members for the potential decisions that lie ahead, offering available alternatives such as the use of opioids to reduce the distress of dyspnoea. If no preparation has been possible through discussion of levels 1–3 (above), an acute crisis of hypoventilation with dyspnoea or retained secretions will often pre-empt decision-making by leading to emergency intervention, even immediate tracheostomy.

After assisted ventilation has been initiated via a tracheostomy, the disease may progress to a stage where communication becomes quite impossible (as in locked-in syndrome), allowing no opportunity to discuss the withdrawal of ventilation support. Where the law does not allow withdrawal of life-sustaining treatments, there may be reluctance to introduce a tracheostomy even for cleaning secretions (level 3, above) because it may be seen to lead inevitably to long-term ventilation.

COUGH

Cough is a protective mechanism, a reflex automatic response or a voluntary movement usually triggered by stimulation of bronchial receptors. Air is held behind closed vocal cords and pressure built up with expiratory muscles, and then suddenly released. A major problem in neuromuscular disease is failure to cough effectively, leading to retention of secretions, and vulnerability to chest infection.

Cough operates appropriately in smokers, or in diseases such as bronchitis, by expelling excess mucus. Cough occurring with lying down may be due to reflux and aspiration of gastric content. In other conditions there may be a dry, persistent cough producing no sputum and caused by sensitivity of the bronchi to cold air, or inhaled particles or chemicals. Such a cough can be exhausting.

Assistance with coughing

Ineffective cough in neuromuscular disease is commonly associated with the accumulation of thick mucous secretions difficult to expel. Inhaled bronchodilatator medications may help give some relief to some patients:

- *salbutamol 2.5, 5 mg/2.5 ml* or *ipratropium 250, 500 µg/ml* by inhaler up to qid.

Helping to fill the lungs by assisting inspiration with a mask and bag as a prelude to a cough can be helpful. Brisk abdominal or lower chest compression timed to coincide with the expiratory effort may assist the cough of a weakened individual. Cough respirators mechanically assist coughing and may be suggested when the peak cough flow rate (in a respiratory flow study) falls below 270 l/min.

Suppression of cough

Opioids are the most satisfactory cough suppressants, using either one of the 'weaker' opioids as mixtures containing codeine, pholcodeine or dextromethorphan; or morphine, diamorphine, oxycodone or hydromorphone in oral or injected forms. Oral morphine suspension 5–10 mg can be used every few hours, and controlled-release preparations may also prove useful in similar small doses.

A persistent, exhausting dry cough may be more effectively suppressed by adding an inhaled local anaesthetic to salbutamol or ipratropium in a nebulizer:

- *2 ml of 1% lignocaine* up to qid.

RETAINED SECRETIONS

The accumulation of thick sticky secretions in the upper airways irritates the bronchi and is difficult to remove if cough is inadequate. Suction cannot reach the sites of accumulation (except via a tracheostomy) and attempts are uncomfortable. The secretions may be made easier to expel if thinned by nebulized saline delivered via mask and air pump, and inhaled salbutamol may be added if there is associated reflex broncho-constriction. Assisted expiration is helpful, and vibration massage to the chest may help mobilize the secretions and make then easier to expel. The enzymes in papaya are sometimes recommended in seeking to make oral mucus thinner; for deeper levels in the respiratory tract inhalations of actylcysteine (*Mucomyst*), which is recommended for treatment of cystic fibrosis and bronchiectasis, can have a useful role.

Death rattle

The presence of mucus in the airways or in the pharynx of patients with advanced illness can lead to a regular gurgling sound with each breath. It is common in the terminal stages of many diseases, more often seen in head injury and in unconscious patients. Family members, who find the noise upsetting, need explanation that the noise is not necessarily indicating distress for the patient. It will usually be appropriate to reduce or cease hydration with I-V or S/C fluids, and occasionally the use of a diuretic (frusemide 20–40 mg I-V) will reduce noisy breathing, suggesting an element of pulmonary congestion. When there are secretions in the pharynx, they may be reduced by anticholinergic drugs:

- *glycopyrrolate 0.2 mg/ml;*
- *atropine 0.6 mg/ml;*
- *hyoscine hydrobromide 0.4 mg/ml.*

These are administered S/C every few hours or as a total of three or four such doses given via a continuous infusion over 24 h. These medications will dry pharyngeal secretions, but will not be as effective for excess secretions in the bronchi.

5

Gastrointestinal symptoms

DRY MOUTH

A dry and painful mouth diminishes quality of life for patients with a terminal illness. Simple measures to relieve this discomfort can result in improved appetite, easier eating and enhance the sense of well-being.

Thirst is a complex symptom with many contributory causes. Adequate management of dry mouth and close attention to mouth care can significantly reduce the discomfort of thirst.

Dehydration is one factor in dry mouth and thirst; others include mouth breathing, increased respiratory effort, diminished saliva production and medications (tricyclic antidepressants, antihistamines and anticholinergics may all contribute).

Some patients with bulbar symptoms are still able to lift a cup to moisten the mouth. If not, spraying the mouth with plain water from a plastic bottle or atomizer gives good relief.

Careful and repeated mouth toilets assist comfort, and involve:

- mouthwashes every few hours with sodium bicarbonate solution or plain water;
- analgesic gels or liquids to counter-act pain from ulceration;
- cleaning away of debris with moist swab-sticks;
- gentle brushing of the teeth;
- encouragement of saliva flow with fresh pineapple pieces, frozen lemon slices, frozen tonic water or chewing gum, plus frequent sips from a feeding cup, syringe or on a soaked swab.

Artificial saliva is not always valuable; mouth washes containing alcohol can increase the dryness. Lip dryness and cracking adds to the discomfort of dry mouth and is assisted by frequent, thin applications of petroleum jelly.

Pilocarpine 1–4% solution (as available in eyedrops, and introduced as a few drops into the mouth) has a limited effect in promoting saliva flow, but can also cause side-effects such as delirium.

CANDIDA INFECTION

Yeast infection of the oral cavity can occur in any individual with advanced illness, more frequently in those with deficient immune responses or receiving corticosteroids.

Management with a topical preparation is usually effective:

- *nystatin 10 000 U/ml susp.* 1 ml qid;
- *amphotericin 10 mg lozenge.* 1 qid;
- *miconazole 20 mg/ml gel.* 2–5 ml qid.

Resistant cases may need:

- *fluconazole 50, 100, 150, 200 mg tab.* 100–200 mg daily or
- *ketoconazole 200 mg tab.* 200 mg orally, daily for 10 days.

DYSPHAGIA

See Chapter on Bulbar symptoms of this section, p. 65.

GASTRO–OESOPHAGEAL REFLUX

The valvular mechanism at the junction of oesophagus and stomach is finely tuned and its function of closing to prevent leakage of gastric content is readily disturbed by changes in local anatomy through tumours, ascites, obesity, extreme weight loss or muscle weakness. Although not a major symptom in advanced neurological conditions, it is a cause of discomfort. Elevation of the bedhead, stopping smoking and suspending the use of non-steroidal anti-inflammatory drugs (NSAIDs) contribute to relief of symptoms.

Regular therapy with non-absorbable antacids:

- *magnesium hydroxide + aluminium hydroxide susp.* 10–20 ml orally, prn,

neutralizes acid leaking up from the stomach.

A histamine H_2-receptor antagonist, for example:

- *cimetidine 200, 400, 800 mg tab.*;
- *famotidine 20, 40 mg tab.*;
- *ranitidine 150, 300 mg tab,*

once or twice daily as required, will reduce gastric acid production.

For patients with persistent symptoms, ongoing treatment aims to ensure comfort, heal oesophagitis if present, and prevent complications. A proton pump inhibitor (PPI) taken daily usually effects a rapid response, but needs to be continued for several weeks:

- *omeprazole 20 mg cap.;*
- *pantoprazole 20, 40 mg tab.; 40 mg inj.;*
- *esomeprazole 20, 40 mg tab.;*
- *lansoprazole 15, 30 mg cap.; 30 mg granules;*
- *rabeprazole 20 mg tab.*

NAUSEA AND VOMITING

A wide variety of stimuli at the vomiting centre activate a neuromuscular reflex – a complex common pathway involving abdominal muscles and viscera, gastric contraction, hypersalivation and sometimes disturbances of cardiac rhythm.

There are many causes of such stimulation: motion sickness, vestibular disturbances, intracranial pathology, pregnancy, gastroenteritis, medication side-effects, metabolic disturbances, radiotherapy or after surgery. Many receptor sites are involved in the emetic response (dopamine D_2, histamine H_1, 5-hydroxytryptamine (5-HT) and muscarinic cholinergic). No anti-emetic agent antagonizes all the receptor sites. Understanding the cause and the likelihood of adverse effects will assist the choice of an appropriate anti-emetic.

In neurological diseases, high spinal injuries or quadriplegia may lead to gastric stasis, particularly in the early phase following injury. Gastroparesis also occurs in longstanding diabetes and other types of autonomic neuropathy, chronic renal failure, dermatomyositis, polymyositis and myotonic dystrophy (in which smooth muscle of the gut may be affected, leading to a motility disorder). Patients will prefer small, frequent meals.

Drug treatments are not very effective, and basic antiemetics are the first choice.

- *metoclopramide 10 mg tab.* 5–10 mg;
- *domperidone 10 mg tab.* 10–20 mg,

orally prior to meals three to four times daily.

Increased intracranial pressure from tumour or infection may stimulate the emetic centre in the floor of the fourth ventricle:

- *cyclizine 50 mg tab.; inj.* up to 150 mg/24 h, plus
- *dexamethasone 4 mg tab.; 4–8 mg inj.* up to 16 mg/24 h

may be more effective.

Some clinicians prefer ondansetron or other members of the family of 5-HT$_3$ antagonists.

Activation of the vestibular system through motion, Meniere's disease or labyrinthitis responds better to anticholinergic and antihistamine drugs:

- *dimenhydrinate 25, 50 mg tab.* 50–100 mg orally, 4–6 hourly, up to 400 mg/24 h;
- *hyoscine hydrobromide 300 μg tab.* 300–600 μg orally, 4–6 hourly, up to 1200 μg/24 h;
- *promethazine hydrochloride 10, 25 mg tab.; 5 mg/5 ml susp.* 8–12 hourly, up to 100 mg/24 h.

Nausea and vomiting is predictably associated with cytotoxic therapy such as cisplatin, either very soon after the therapy or during the days following. After radiation therapy, nausea and vomiting are not as predictable or severe and may require no specific therapy:

- *metoclopramide 10–20 mg subcutaneous (S/C)* may be effective for minor nausea and vomiting, given prior to the treatment and for several days following.

Where severe vomiting is anticipated use:

- *ondansetron 8 mg inj., tab.* oral or S/C tds ac or
- *tropisetron 5 mg inj., tab.* oral or S/C tds ac, together with a single dose of
- *dexamethasone 8 mg inj., tab.* S/C or intravenous (I-V) inj.

Many other drugs can cause nausea and vomiting: dopamine agonists, levodopa (L-dopa), bromocriptine and opioids. Opioids have a direct effect on the emetic centre in the third ventricle, and also slow gastric emptying. Where possible, reduce the dose of the offending drug, or change to a different formulation.

Vomiting occurs in gastroenteritis, but no anti-emetic treatment should be required, the emphasis being on maintaining hydration.

Nausea and vomiting may also be a learned response, as in the anticipatory nausea associated with chemotherapy, or related to anxiety, a bad smell or disgusting sight.

Hyperacidity may produce considerable nausea, heartburn, acidity or bitter taste. The use of antacids, histamine H_2-receptor antagonists (cimetidine, ranitidine, famotidine) or a PPI such as omeprazole 20 mg orally will be effective.

Mucosal erosion secondary to NSAID use may be associated with significant nausea. Protection for the stomach mucosa is provided by:

- *misoprostol 200 μg tab.* two to four times daily or
- *omeprazole 20 mg tab.* up to 80 mg once daily.

A common cause of occasional nausea to be kept in mind for neurological disease is constipation (v.i.).

Vomiting that occurs suddenly with no or very little nausea raises suspicion of upper gastrointestinal obstruction or intracranial disease.

Anti-emetic medications

Prochlorperazine and haloperidol have antipsychotic as well as anti-emetic properties:

- *prochlorperazine 5 mg tab. 25 mg suppository* is given up to tds orally or bd rectally;
- *haloperidol 0.5, 1.5, 5 mg tab.; 5, 10 mg/ml inj.* have the advantage of being available for S/C administration either as a bolus of 0.5–2.5 mg or up to 15 mg/24 h in a continuous infusion.

Acute extrapyramidal reactions are uncommon but may occur with either drug, and this class is best avoided in Parkinson's disease.

Cyclizine is one of the most popular anti-emetics used in the UK, with its principal action at the vomiting centre:

- *cyclizine 50 mg tab.; 50 mg/ml inj.* 25–50 mg tds, up to 150 mg S/C infusion/24 h.

Metoclopramide and domperidone stimulate motility of the upper gastrointestinal tract, increasing gastric emptying rate and reducing small intestinal transit time in doses of 10–20 mg tds. Metoclopramide is an antagonist at dopamine receptors in the central nervous system and can produce sedation and other extrapyramidal adverse effects. The most important of these adverse effects are the acute dystonic and dysphoric reactions, sometimes severe (e.g. oculogyric crisis), and more common in children and young adults:

- *metoclopramide 10 mg tab.; 10 mg/2 ml inj.* up to 80 mg/24 h.

Acute dystonic reactions should be treated with:

- *benzhexol 2, 5 mg tab.* up to 5 mg once daily or bd or
- *benztropine 2 mg tab.; 2 mg/ml inj.* 2 mg once daily or bd.

Side effects limit their use in older persons.

Like prochlorperazine, metoclopramide has additive sedative effects with alcohol, benzodiazepines, opioids and other central nervous system depressants.

Domperidone is also a dopamine antagonist, but does not readily cross the blood–brain barrier and therefore is less likely to cause acute extrapyramidal (dystonic) reactions. Unlike metoclopramide it is not readily available as an injection. Adverse effects include mild abdominal cramps, dry mouth and galactorrhoea:

- *domperidone 10 tab.* up to 80 mg/24 h.

Ondansetron and other H_2-receptor antagonists are commonly reserved for protection against vomiting due to cytotoxic drugs, and given once before each chemotherapy, but may have a place as second line drugs for persistent nausea and vomiting (but considerably more expensive):

- *ondansetron 4, 8 mg tab.; 4, 8 mg inj.; 4 mg oral wafer, 4 mg/5 ml susp., 16 mg suppository;*
- *tropisetron 5 mg cap.; 1 mg/ml inj.* 5 mg orally or I-V;
- *dolestron 50, 200 mg tab.; 20 mg/ml inj.* 200 mg orally or 100 mg I-V daily.

BOWEL DYSFUNCTION

What is regarded as normal bowel function varies greatly, and for any patient what is normal for that individual should first be clarified. The process of defaecation depends partly on sensory awareness (detecting stool in the rectum) and also on motor control, requiring relaxation of the anal sphincters and pelvic floor muscles and contraction of the abdominal wall and diaphragm. The delivery of bowel content to the lower colon is assisted by parasympathetic innervation that may be disturbed in spinal or pelvic disease.

Constipation

Reduction in fluid intake, lack of privacy, change in diet, lack of exercise, slowed transit of bowel content and weakened muscles of chest, abdomen and pelvic floor, all of which are common in advanced neurological diseases such as amyotrophic lateral sclerosis (ALS) or multiple sclerosis (MS), contribute to a dry hard stool that is difficult to pass.

More specific nerve damage may also induce constipation. Interruption of the parasympathetic nerve supply to the colon (as in low spinal lesions) may inhibit normal peristaltic activity and leave a dilated baggy colon. Many of the medications used for symptom management delay bowel transit times (opioids being most consistent in this regard).

Notoriously, constipation makes any other symptom worse.

In healthy individuals, constipation is managed through changing to a diet that contains adequate bulk and fluids, assisted by exercise and the establishment of a regular routine, which can take advantage of the gastric–colic reflex that initiates colon peristalsis following a meal. In persons affected by neurological disorders this approach may still be possible.

An adequate dietary fibre intake (30 g/day) is based on plant complex carbohydrates that escape digestion in the small intestine to be broken down by bacterial enzymes in the large intestine, increasing solid residue and water content in the stool, making them softer, wetter and easier to pass. Bulking agents include wholegrain or wholemeal products (breads, cereals, pastas and rice), fruits and vegetables, legumes, seeds and nuts. Fluid intake must be adequate (2 l/day if possible).

Bulk-forming agents may not be effective in the presence of poor mobility and muscle power, and for many individuals with neurological disease, a laxative will be necessary.

There are three major classes of laxatives (aperients):

- *softeners* that draw additional water into the bowel lumen;
- *sliders* that wet the stool surface or oil its transit;
- *pushers* that stimulate bowel wall contraction.

Stool softeners are osmotic agents, and may be administered up to three times a day:

- *sorbitol 70% liquid* 10–30 ml;
- *lactulose susp.* 10–30 ml;
- *magnesium oxide powder* 5–15 g (one to three teaspoonsful) in water orally;
- *macrogol 13 g sachet* dissolved in 150 ml water. 1–3 sachets.

Paraffin oil that assists stool sliding has been largely abandoned. Docusate is a wetting agent that is also a stool softener; it is often combined with a 'pusher', a bowel stimulant such as:

- *docusate 50 mg + senna 8 mg tab.* two tablets or
- *docusate 120 mg* two tablets + *bisacodyl 5 mg* two tablets, taken orally any evening the bowels have not opened that day, and up to two to three times daily if necessary.

A common regimen will be to start with two tablets of docusate + senna at night if bowels have not been open that day, increasing as necessary to twice daily or three times daily, then adding an osmotic agent such as sorbitol or macrogol up to three times a day.

Many patients prefer natural or herbal preparations, for example prune juice, dried fig preparations or senna 8% with dried fruits 10 g orally, daily at night. Some may contain stimulants such as cascara.

However, when constipation is resistant to increased doses of laxatives, there should be a re-evaluation of the underlying cause(s), including impaction. A rectal examination may discover a bulky stool mass or soft stool in a ballooned rectum that weak muscles cannot expel. A glycerine suppository rectally (allowed to remain for 15 to 30 min) may assist, or a micro enema with sodium citrate (content of 1 tube). If necessary, repeated glycerine and olive oil enemas may be required.

If stool has formed a quite hard mass it will often be best to disimpact it manually under a light anaesthetic administered prior to the procedure:

- *morphine (2.5–5 mg) + midazolam (2.5–5 mg)* I-V bolus, then breaking up the mass with the gloved index finger, and lifting it out through the anus a piece at a time.

Bowel incontinence and diarrhoea

A conscious awareness of distension of the rectum and of its content as gas, liquid or solid allows evacuation to be controlled and timed. Even if the rectal sphincters are normal, lack of sensitivity to distension may result in an accumulation of rectal content without any adequate signal for emptying of the bowel. Changes in the consistency of bowel content, loss of sensation in the perineum and anus, and loss of strength in pelvic and abdominal musculature will all interfere with control.

Faecal incontinence has many causes – abnormal volume and consistency of stool arriving at the rectum, bowel inflammation, anatomical derangement (prolapse, pelvic tumour), damage to the nervous system at many levels, muscle weakness, behavioural abnormalities and dementia. Disabled individuals may have difficulty in observing adequate standards of hygiene, and in institutional settings as well as homes, infectious diarrhoea can cause dramatic incontinence. Giardia infection may be indicated by bulky soft stool with a very offensive odour, and if suspected should be checked by stool microscopy and treated with either:

- *tinidazole 500 mg tab.* 2 g orally, as a single dose or
- *metronidazole 200, 400 mg tab.* 2 g orally, daily for 3 days.

A common problem in the bedfast patient is that constipation causes accumulation of impacted stool in the rectum with leakage of liquid faeces around it, giving the impression of incontinence.

Assessment of diarrhoea and incontinence will review possible causes, perineal sensation, anal reflex and sphincter tone. Digital examination will ensure that there is no impacted mass in the rectum. Its absence does not eliminate accumulation of bowel content higher in the colon. A hard 'brick' of stool in the rectum, may require manual assistance, breaking up the mass with a gloved finger and extracting it in pieces. If perineal sensation is intact, this will prove very painful, and the use of local lignocaine gel plus a light bedside anaesthetic (as above) will make the procedure painless.

In the absence of impaction, diarrhoea not due to infection may resolve with the use of:

- *loperamide 2 mg tab.* up to 8/day or
- *codeine 30 mg tab.* 30–60 mg up to three times daily.

Urine and bowel management in spinal injury

Whereas previous measures for urinary management in paraplegia included resection of the bladder neck and the use of an indwelling catheter, recent routines rely more on regular self-catheterization. The patient will often sense bladder fullness with a slight sweating or other subjective feeling, and with careful sterile technique will avoid introducing infection.

Regular evacuation of the lower bowel is an important routine for individuals living with paraplegia. The stimulation of evacuation is accomplished by taking advantage of basic bowel reflexes (e.g. the gastro-colic reflex that initiates emptying after a meal) and exploring other mechanisms for stimulating evacuation such as the insertion of a glycerine suppository or digital stimulation of the anal canal, in a context of scrupulous adherence to a routine that 'educates' the bowel.

NUTRITION AND HYDRATION

Food and health, well-being and close personal relationships are tied closely together in most cultural settings. When an individual is unable to eat normally, family members feel great concern, and in advanced and terminal illness may hold and express a desperate hope that if the patient could only eat better, some improvement might be achieved. 'If he does not eat, he will die' is a frequently heard expression of concern. To refuse food suggests a rejection of the care being provided or of life itself. Patients who cannot find satisfaction in eating feel life is hardly worthwhile; carers feel they are failing in their duty.

Anorexia

There are many reasons why food intake is reduced in illness. Weakness or paresis causes difficulty in transferring food or drink to the mouth; appetite falls away when infection, tumour or metabolic upset is present; or when taste is altered by drug therapies. A dry or painful mouth inhibits chewing and weakness makes the effort of eating a burden. Difficulty in swallowing leads to aspiration of ingested fluids or foods into the respiratory passages and a fear of choking. Oesophageal atony, obstruction or the reflux of gastric content interferes with the passage of food to the stomach. Nausea, that makes an individual unable to face food, is caused by abdominal or central nervous system pathology predominantly, but also a diverse range of upsets, including unwelcome sights, smells, drugs or constipation.

Nutritional support

In advanced neurological disease, sitting up to swallow may become difficult, and involuntary movements, weakness, swallowing difficulties or fatigue inhibit self-feeding and require patient, slow assistance by carers. Nausea, vomiting, constipation, pain or medications can alter taste and erode appetite.

In the supportive phase of a chronic progressive illness it will be important to encourage an adequate and balanced food intake as part of maintaining comfort and function. Patient preference is the best guide to what should be offered.

Attention to the presentation, flavour and consistency of meals, their timing and setting within a supportive social environment, the posture for receiving and swallowing mouthfuls, and the utensils being used for feeding can all help if there is lack of taste and appetite.

Many drugs alter taste or cause nausea, and a review of appetite in relation to when particular medications were begun may allow offending items to be ceased or a substitute suggested.

Progestational drugs such as:

- *megestrol acetate 40, 160 mg tab.* 160 mg/daily, or
- *medroxyprogesterone acetate 400 mg* daily have a beneficial effect on appetite;
- *cyproheptadine 4 mg tab.* 4 mg up to tds is also used;
- *cannabis,* either smoked or in the form of tablets or cakes and biscuits promotes appetite and well-being in some individuals, particularly if they have used it previously for recreational purposes.

In advanced cancer, corticosteroids will often increase appetite and a sense of well-being:

- *dexamethasone 4 mg tab.* 4 mg with the morning meal, reducing gradually to no more than 1 mg to avoid untoward side-effects – proximal myopathy, hypomania, diabetes, etc.).

Enteral nutrition support (I-V or gastrointestinal tube feeding) is commonly initiated for patients who cannot be fed satisfactorily by mouth. If the gastrointestinal tract remains functional, feeding via a naso-gastric tube or gastrostomy is more practical than I-V parenteral nutrition.

A tube via the nasal route is a source of persistent discomfort, and a gastrostomy or jejunostomy is commonly preferred when enteral nutrition will be needed for longer than a few weeks. Aspiration pneumonia is a serious complication of enteral feeding, whether by nasogastric tube or per-endoscopic gastrostomy (PEG), and bed-bound patients who are sedated are most at risk.

Patients in whom a gastrostomy is inserted may experience diarrhoea, constipation, nausea, vomiting, bloating and gastro-oesophageal reflux. The gastrostomy tube and its attachments may form a focus for bacterial infection, the formula may be contaminated or too hypertonic or delivered too fast and cause diarrhoea; the absence of fibre may induce constipation; nausea or bloating may require a slowing of the infusion rate; reflux may occur if the patient lies too flat (with a risk of aspiration).

Enteral feeding should be considered as primarily a short-term measure for those persons in whom improvement is anticipated or hoped for (e.g. acute stroke, head injury). There is little hard evidence that PEG or nasogastric feeding, used on a permanent basis, improves survival. Therefore it must be questioned whether this method of providing nutrition should be initiated in dementia, established stroke, advanced MS or ALS. Repeated discussion with family members may be necessary to achieve some common decision about whether to continue feeding at all, and if so, by what method.

Withdrawing nutritional support

When some artificial measure to maintain nutrition has been started, it may prove quite difficult to deliberately withdraw it. Families may feel that it is unacceptable to cease feeding, because the patient will 'starve to death'. Therefore the question of *stopping* naso-gastric, gastrostomy or parenteral feeding should be touched upon before such a measure is started. It may be offered as a way of improving the patient's comfort and well-being, or tiding a situation over in anticipation of spontaneous recovery or improvement following other therapy, with the warning that if those outcomes are not achieved, it will be appropriate to cease the artificial method of providing nutrition. This issue is discussed further in the section on Ethics under the heading Persistent Vegetative State (p. 209).

Family members may need to be reassured that any suggestion of discomfort that might follow stopping the provision of calories and protein will be treated promptly with medications that address pain and restlessness effectively. Often a continuous 24 h S/C infusion with:

- *morphine 5–10 mg + midazolam 5–10 mg* will be sufficient.

Hydration

Whereas patients who lose appetite will commonly not feel hungry, the inability to maintain a satisfactory fluid intake can induce thirst and postural hypotension. If the patient who is unable to swallow fluids in sufficient volume to maintain hydration complains of thirst or is perceived to suffer thirst, regular ice chips by mouth and frequent mouth care will assist comfort (p. 77).

If additional fluids are to be administered, I-V normal saline or dextrose 4% in 1/5 N saline will counter dehydration in a hospital setting, but I-V fluids are not so readily administered in home settings. Here the continuous S/C infusion of 1 l of fluid (saline or dextrose/saline) over 24 h (hypodermoclysis) is available. Via a plastic S/C cannula (e.g. 'Intima') inserted into the S/C tissues over the pectoral area, the anterior abdominal wall or thigh, 1 l of fluid (saline or dextrose/saline), run in over 24 h, will be slowly absorbed and is usually tolerated on a continuous basis. The site of infusion should be changed every 2 or 3 days. Whether it alters prognosis, however, is doubtful, unless the situation being managed is short term and improvement is anticipated.

Withdrawal of such attempts at maintaining adequate hydration is not commonly accompanied by a symptom of thirst when an individual is in the closing phase of an illness, and provided mouth care is continued, family members can be reassured that the body becoming dry is a component of the natural dying process. It contributes to gentle sedation, it reduces the need to pass urine, and it does not cause any major discomfort.

6

Urological symptoms

Urinary symptoms may be primarily irritative, obstructive or both. Hyperreflexia leads to urgency, frequency and incontinence, and frequent bladder spasms. Hesitancy leads on to retention of urine and overflow incontinence. The aim of management is to establish the ability to retain an adequate volume of urine at low pressure in the bladder, and an acceptable routine for voiding. Long-term follow-up for patients with neurogenic bladder problems will aim to preserve renal function and avoid infections by promoting continence, acceptable bladder storage and controlled emptying while minimizing symptoms in a manner that promotes improved quality of life and self-esteem.

Some common urinary symptoms result from local pathology:

• urinary infection,
• vaginal wall atrophy or prolapse,
• bladder tumours,
• prostatic hypertrophy or malignancy or
• abdominal pathology.

When neurological disorders compromise bladder control, the primary symptoms depend on the level and type of damage to the nervous system.

Incontinence is common following a stroke, due to involuntary bladder wall contraction. This may also be seen in Parkinson's disease, and in multiple sclerosis (MS). Spinal cord lesions above the level of the sacral innervation cause an initial retention of urine that may be followed by overflow incontinence and later a reflex involuntary pattern of voiding. Lower spinal lesions result in a bladder unable to contract.

Pelvic nerve damage (e.g. from diabetic neuropathy or pelvic surgery) may destroy sensations of bladder fullness and cause retention and overflow incontinence.

The assessment of urological discomfort demands a comprehensive history of the underlying disease(s), plus a description of voiding difficulties and a careful examination to establish mental status, neurological deficits and the presence of any local pathology. Urodynamic investigation allows more specific definition of micturition disturbances to guide therapeutic decisions.

URINARY RETENTION

Patients seek both comfort and control, if possible without surgical intervention or the use of catheters. Prostatic hypertrophy is the commonest cause of urinary difficulty in older males, and may complicate the effect of nerve damage associated with an overactive detrusor muscle, hesitancy and inability to empty the bladder. High post-void residual bladder volumes (PVR, normally only a few millilitres) – are a common finding and increase the risk of bacterial infection. To lessen this, patients are encouraged to undertake regular bladder emptying, employing double voiding that may need to be assisted by abdominal pressure. Prompt recognition and treatment of infection is desirable, and prophylactic antibiotics may be indicated.

Alpha-1 blocking drugs (prazosin, or long-acting formulations terazosin or tasulosin) may decrease PVR volumes in male patients with prostatic hypertrophy in whom surgery is unwise. Where obstruction to flow, or retention of urine from other causes (e.g. spinal injury) is established, intermittent self-catheterization is preferable to an indwelling catheter, but will be beyond the capacity of many elderly individuals or patients with neurological disorders. For some female patients self-catheterization is also quite difficult. If infections recur, there may be adequate suppression of bacteria with:

- *hexamine hippurate 1 g tab.* + *vitamin C 500 mg tab.* bd–qid.

Alternating treatment with:

- *trimethoprim 300 mg tab.* daily and
- *nitrofuradantin 50 mg tab.* daily is also suggested.

An indwelling catheter draining into a leg bag (strapped to the calf) allows movement and sitting out in a chair. The strap sometimes increases local muscle spasm, the bag must be below the level of the bladder, and not allowed to become overfull.

Indwelling catheters inevitably cause a urinary infection, and there is often persistent discomfort from bladder spasm or bladder neck irritation, for which antispasmodic drugs such as oxybutynin 2.5–5 mg tds may give some relief. Indications for using an indwelling catheter include protection of local skin from maceration and ulceration, overflow incontinence when obstruction cannot be relieved by surgery, difficulty in making frequent changes of soiled pads or clothing, and when the illness is regarded as terminal. Catheters for indwelling use should be small (French size 14) and silicone or teflon coated, with a small retention balloon of 10 ml, and drain into a closed bag. Catheters may commonly be left in place for up to 2 months; encrustation is common; leakage may indicate constipation and a full rectum, or bladder infection.

When bladder drainage will be necessary over a long period of time (as in MS) it is best achieved via a permanent supra-pubic catheter which allows freer drainage and a reduced risk of infection.

URGENCY AND BLADDER SPASM

Damage to the innervation of the bladder may lead to urgency, urge incontinence and bladder spasms. Improved control may result from avoiding caffeine, and monitoring fluid intake in advance of times when opportunity to pass urine is restricted; other non-drug treatments include pelvic floor training and the use of biofeedback techniques:

- *oxybutynin 5 mg tab.* 10–20 mg/day, or
- *propantheline 15 mg tab.* 45–90 mg/day reduce the strength and frequency of bladder wall contractions.

A controlled-release formulation of oxybutynin is available in some countries and can be effective in a single daily dose. An alternative approach instils capsaicin into the bladder cavity, and the use of botulinum toxin by the same route has a longer-lasting effect, but is not widely available.

Frequency may be reduced by tricyclic antidepressants, for example:

- *imipramine 25 mg tab.* 25–75 mg at night.

The vasopressin analogue, desmopressin may be given by intranasal insufflation before sleep and reduces the accumulation of urine during the night:

- *desmopressin 10 μg/spray.*

Self-catheterization is practised successfully by some patients, but for others a better solution may be an implanted bladder stimulator or permanent drainage via a supra-pubic drain rather than a urinary catheter.

Electrical stimulation, an intrusive and expensive procedure, will inhibit micturition when applied to the hypogastric plexus (originating from spinal levels Th10-L2) and encourage voiding by stimulation of sympathetic nerves.

URINARY INCONTINENCE

Incontinence of urine is a frequent cause of embarrassment and discomfort. As a basis for other strategies of treatment, regular times for voiding and fluid restriction prior to public occasions should be practised. Antispasmodic drugs will assist control. Imipramine 25–50 mg at night or bd increases bladder outlet resistance. Tricyclic antidepressants are a cause of retention of urine in males, but may assist incontinence in females.

- *dicyclomine 10 mg tab.* 10–40 mg tds reduces bladder contraction but anticholinergic side-effects may be severe;
- *nifedipine 10 mg tab.* up to tds has been suggested for reduction of urge incontinence.

Surgical manoeuvres such as periurethral collagen injection or pubovaginal sling operations have little place in neurological disorders.

Considerable assistance may be found from the incontinence nurse, who can teach simple strategies and encourage other staff in prompting patients regularly when it is time to void, and in encouraging fluid restriction.

The use of external collection devices draining to a bedside bag is a common measure.

Condom drains for males require careful preparation if they are not to become dislodged. The penile skin should be clean and dry and the pubic hair clipped or shaved. Other (less practical) attachments have been marketed for women.

Absorbent pads held in place with net briefs are a welcome alternative to soiled underwear; inserts may have a pocket shape to accommodate the penis. Disposable diapers are commonly used, and absorbent underpads will protect bedding and chairs, having a waterproof backing to a layer of absorbent material under a soft permeable cover against the skin. The problem of acid urine irritating skin prone to pressure ulceration remains, and meticulous skin care with regular cleansing and prompt treatment of rashes, excoriated areas or thrush infection is mandatory. Barrier creams and other water-soluble moisturizers are a helpful addition to skin care.

Penile clamps need careful supervision and regular release every 2–4 h, and are therefore often inappropriate for patients with impaired cognition or dexterity. Monilia infection commonly becomes established in areas frequently soiled with urine, and is recognized by the bright red 'scalded' appearance of the skin:

- *clotrimazole 1%, miconazole 2% or bifanazole 1% creams* are quickly effective, but reinfection is common.

SEXUAL DYSFUNCTION

Satisfactory sexual function depends on a complex relationship between the individual and that person's intimate human context and cultural environment. Parasympathetic, sympathetic and somatosensory nerve integrity may all be required for a coordinated physiological response to sexual stimulation and it is readily impaired by central or peripheral neurological disorder. In the male, erectile dysfunction may be anticipated after radical retropubic prostatectomy, spinal cord injury or any chronic neurological disease. In diabetic men, erectile dysfunction is associated with autonomic neuropathy.

Drugs that may inhibit attaining a satisfactory erection include oestrogens (used in the treatment of prostatic cancer), antihypertensive and cardiac drugs; phenothiazines, antidiabetic agents and tricyclic antidepressants.

It is often difficult for patients to reveal distress caused by loss of sexual satisfaction, and it can be accompanied by hidden emotions of loss, guilt and anger. When sexual dysfunction is suspected, a gentle exploration by the clinician may be met with a grateful response by the patient, but that approach may also be quickly rejected. Any treatment undertaken should begin with the least invasive methods and involve both partners where practicable in a whole-patient approach, exploring sexual need and satisfaction for both.

In MS a reduced libido and failure to attain orgasm is frequent in both men and women, with decreased vaginal lubrication in women, and impotence, erectile dysfunction and failure of ejaculation in men. Symptoms of depression and anxiety may be recognized and contribute to sexual dysfunction. Women may experience painful perineal dysaesthesia or diminished sensation. Premature ejaculation generally responds to selective serotonin re-uptake inhibitors such as paroxetine. Corticosteroid treatment given for other reasons has been found to improve sexual function in some individuals.

Treatment of erection failure in conditions such as MS depended on injection of papaverine intra-corporeally into the penis, until the advent of sildenafil, an inhibitor of the enzyme phosphodiesterase type 5:

- *Sildenafil 25 mg tab.* Two taken 1 h before sexual activity encourages a satisfactory penile erection in a majority of males.

Sildenafil is now supplemented by apomorphine SL, a dopamine D_1- and D_2-receptor agonist, and vardenafil and tadalafil, new phosphodiesterase type 5 inhibitors. Side effects of sildenafil include flushing, headache, dyspepsia and visual disturbances but the use of this medication has not been associated with serious cardiovascular events or death. Patients who do not respond to phosphodiesterase inhibitors may employ intracavernosal or intraurethral therapy with alprostadil. Research in female sexual dysfunction has led to no interventions comparable to what has been developed for males. Nevertheless, women are likely to welcome the opportunity to discuss their problem.

Sexual activity entails much more than genital penetration, and encouragement to engage in cuddling, stroking, kissing and other forms of intimate exchange may provide acceptable levels of satisfaction for many couples for whom one partner is suffering neurological impairment. To see a partner climb onto a hospital bed to hold a life mate in a close and loving embrace is a moving experience, and an appropriate action. Such intimacy should be not only allowed but encouraged and facilitated.

Pain is often the most feared symptom of disease. Palliative care, through its major experience with cancer, has developed a primary expertise in the assessment and management of pain. In neurological conditions pain is a surprisingly common feature but is often less precisely described, and may be less easily assessed and managed.

TYPES AND MECHANISMS OF PAIN

The physiological and pathological mechanisms underlying an experience of pain are very complex. Recent research has begun to clarify the plasticity of response to stimulation that is characteristic of nerve tissue, and its susceptibility to hyperexcitability with the induction of pain in areas away from the initial site of damage to tissue. The dynamic and flexible nature of nervous system function defies simple classification and explanation. Nevertheless, it remains useful to distinguish two major types of pain.

Nociceptive. Where cell damage is caused by trauma, pressure, heat or cold and there is an associated inflammatory response that stimulates specialized nerve endings (nociceptors), with impulses conducted centrally to initiate an experience of pain. That pain can usually be localized to the site of the stimulus, and is experienced either as a sharp discomfort, an ache or a sensation of pressure or tightness, and may be relieved with common analgesics including opioids.

It is important that such pain stimulation from a site of injury be not visualized as a simple cascade of ascending impulses within the nervous system. Stimulation is conducted widely, with many associated relevant effects (physical and emotional), and descending impulses are also evoked simultaneously, and will moderate and modify the pain experience.

Neuropathic. Where nerve tissue is directly affected (by trauma, pressure, infarction, etc.) pain is experienced in the region served by those neurones or their connections, but is poorly localized, and commonly is reported as having a burning quality, or a feeling of pins and needles, numbness or hypersensitivity in the affected area, or unheralded sudden shooting pains. Neuropathic pain does not respond so readily to usual forms of analgesia. Although common analgesics still have a place in management, membrane-stabilizing drugs, from within the classes of antidepressants, anticonvulsants or antidysrhythmics, may offer more specific relief.

Each of these two main types of pain can be further divided into sub-types:

Nociceptive pain may follow stimulus of receptors in cutaneous, visceral or musculoskeletal tissues:

- The experience of cutaneous pain is superficial, sharp or burning, and localized around the site of injury.
- Muscle pain is experienced as a diffuse ache, sometimes associated with referred pain and local hyperalgesia.
- Visceral pain is common in cancer, sometimes intermittent if associated with smooth muscle contraction in bowel or other tubal structures.

Neuropathic pain may be subdivided into peripheral nerve injury (as in peripheral neuropathy or amputation) and central pain from injury at the level of spinal cord, thalamus or cerebrum (as from ischaemic stroke).

THE IMPORTANCE OF EARLY CONTROL OF PAIN

Early effective control of pain will minimize progressive excitation of the nervous system. That excitation, if unchecked by treatment, may lead to anatomical changes in dorsal horn neurons and expansion of those changes into surrounding neurones. The clinical result of such changes can be:

- *hyperalgesia* (increased pain response to noxious stimuli);
- *allodynia* (pain experienced with normally innocuous stimuli);
- *spontaneous pain;*
- *referred pain* or
- *sympathetically maintained pain.*

All are undesirable consequences and difficult to manage.

'Pain memory' may be an important part of the pain experience, and has led to the promotion of pre-emptive analgesia, administering analgesics prior to a noxious stimulus or injury (e.g. a surgical operation). Clinical trials of such an approach have had mixed results, however. What is well accepted is that pain needs to be promptly and adequately treated. Left untreated, pain will become worse, and will be more difficult to control.

PAIN IN NEUROLOGY

The neurology patient faces some particular pain issues, including:

- Immobility and pain from muscle stiffness and spasticity.
- Skin pressure soreness and ulceration from immobility, incontinence.
- Interference with expression of pain symptoms through impairment of intellectual function or speech.
- Neuropathic pain from damage to nerve fibres, nerve tracts, and neurones.
- Absence of pain through damage to sensory pathways, leading to an increase in joint damage, skin ulceration, trophic sores, burns and other accidental injury.

Some diseases will present particular challenges:

- Pain in multiple sclerosis (MS) can be acute, arising from ectopic excitation at sites of demyelination; sub-acute (as in bladder spasm or pressure sores); and chronic caused by dysaesthesia in the extremities, or spasm of muscles. Each of these pain types in MS may require a different combination of medications.
- Muscle soreness and stiffness, and skin pressure problems will be common where there is loss of motor function, as in amyotrophic lateral sclerosis (ALS) or muscular dystrophy.
- In cerebral infarction there may initially be no pain, but later a disturbing but poorly localized discomfort may signal central pain.
- In spinal cord disease, a first sign may be girdle pain at level of the pathology.
- Many patients with para- or tetraplegia of traumatic origin suffer from severe, continuous burning and/or lancinating pain. In spinal cord injury there may be a segmentally distributed pain at the level of the lesion; also pain in the body below the lesion, sometimes of late onset, and therefore be easily missed and neglected. In skin or viscera below the level of the lesion the patient may experience allodynia. Partial spinal lesions cause more pain than complete lesions.

- In central pain the intensity of discomfort seems independent of the level of stimulus.
- In peripheral neuropathy or leprosy the absence of pain will lead to trophic ulceration in pressure areas, burns to the extremities, neuropathic joints.

Assessment of pain

'*Pain is what the patient says hurts*' is a statement which emphasizes the need to start assessment with the patient's own account, expanding it with careful attention to the site, timing, character, intensity and review of the measures which either decrease or increase the discomfort caused.

Clearly, in a number of situations familiar to neurologists, either because of dementia or loss of the power of speech, it will be impossible to obtain a clear account of the patient's discomfort. Reliance must be placed on careful observation of non-verbal signs, such as grimacing with movement or avoidance of certain positions or activities. Reports by nurses or family who attend the patient over a period will be particularly useful (see chapter on Dementia, Section III, p. 148).

It will also be important to assess the wider impact that pain is having on patient well-being and on family and social circumstances. The discomfort and limitation imposed by pain affects most activities, and may lead also to depression, despair and anger.

Medications for pain management

Within any comprehensive plan for patient support and the relief of discomfort, the effective relief of pain remains a central concern, and the appropriate use of analgesics stands at the core of pain management.

The World Health Organization (WHO) ladder

World Health Organization (WHO) publications on Cancer Pain Relief have clearly summarized principles of analgesic use that are relevant to the management of all chronic pain. The method recommended is summarized under five headings:

By mouth (using the most convenient routes of administration).

By the clock (using doses at regular intervals, before pain returns; not waiting for a further complaint as though the patient needs to 'earn' the pain medication) by waiting until it becomes really unbearable!

By the ladder The WHO ladder (Figure 11.7.1), with its three levels of mild pain, moderate pain and severe pain, progressive levels being managed

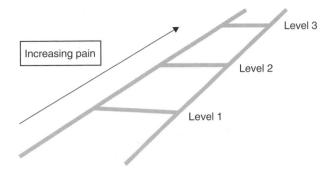

Figure 11.7.1 The WHO pain ladder. Level 1: simple analgesics – aspirin, paracetamol, NSAIDs. Level 2: minor opioids – tramadol, codeine, dextropropoxyphene. Level 3: major opioids – morphine, oxycodone, fentanyl, hydromorphone, diamorphine.

with increasingly potent analgesics and increasing doses, was introduced as a teaching tool.

It embodies an important principle – that there is no best analgesic or correct dose which can be applied to all cases, and the use of increasingly powerful analgesics and an increase in dose must be undertaken until pain is adequately controlled.

There is now wide recognition that the WHO ladder, in its suggestion of a steady increase in type and dose of analgesic, is not always appropriate for severe pain, where an immediate use of major opioids is necessary. Many clinicians, having recognized that simple analgesics (level 1) are ineffective, will move directly to Level 3 drugs. Many will suggest that the term 'minor opioid' is misleading; these are opioids for which high doses will give good pain relief, but side-effects may cause great difficulty at those doses.

For the individual This emphasizes that analgesia must be individualized; there are no standard doses; the only 'right' dose is the one that relieves the patient's pain. This is particularly applicable to the use of opioids. Of the several major opioids that are now available in modern medicine, one or two may suit a particular patient best, and the dose that 'works' may vary from tiny to massive doses.

Attention to detail This refers to the need to document both baseline and break-through doses, and explain to patient, family and staff the recommended regimen, and how to monitor its effectiveness. They should be informed of the side-effects to anticipate, the importance of changing doses if pain escalates, and the need to seek advice to revise the treatment schedule if necessary.

MANAGEMENT OF NOCICEPTIVE PAIN

For any one step on the WHO ladder no particular drug is consistently superior.

At the first step, where non-opioid drugs are employed, there is a choice of aspirin, paracetamol and the range of non-steroidal anti-inflammatory drugs (NSAID), any of which may cause side-effects.

At the second level, it is recommended that non-opioid analgesics be continued, but opioids will be introduced also. Both tramadol and codeine have been regarded as 'weak' opioids, and considered as appropriate to the second level of the ladder, but many clinicians prefer to move directly to one of the major opioids, blurring the distinction between the second and the third level of the ladder:

- *tramadol 50 mg cap., 100, 150 mg sustained-release formulation (SR) tab.; 100, 500 mg inj.* 50–100 mg bd–qid is preferred by some clinicians (especially if there is an element of neuropathic pain); others move directly to major opioid preparations.

Third level opioids include morphine, oxycodone, hydromorphone and fentanyl. Diamorphine remains popular in the UK.

There are, of course, many other opioids on the market, including pethidine (meperidine), buprenorphine, pentazocine, dextromoramide, sufentanyl, and methadone; these are not commonly used in palliative care practice, though sufentanyl and methadone have some special indications. Pethidine, used repeatedly over a period, can lead to accumulation of a metabolite, nor-pethidine, and this has the capacity to cause seizures. Buprenorphine and pentazocine are mixed agonist–antagonist opioids, developed in the hope of diminishing any risk of addiction. This makes them far less suitable to be employed in high doses.

Which of the opioids is preferred will depend on availability, the clinical context, the past experience of the patient and the clinician, and preferred routes of administration.

Where there is renal impairment, fentanyl, which does not depend on renal excretion, may be preferred to morphine. If morphine has previously caused confusion, a change to oxycodone or fentanyl may be beneficial. Fentanyl is also thought to cause less constipation than other opioids.

It is very helpful if clinicians have access to more than one opioid drug, because for any single opioid there will be some individuals who tolerate it poorly, but do well on an alternative. Similarly, for one opioid, there will be a wide variation in response to a particular dose, some opioid-naïve individuals gaining excellent pain control from very small doses, others gaining little relief and finding that higher doses cause unwelcome side-effects.

National regulatory authorities reach different decisions when determining which opioids will be licensed for use, and which formulations will be made available. Oral morphine in solution may be prohibited, but controlled-release preparations allowed; a number of opioids, and particularly injected formulations, may be permitted in hospital practice but not made available for home care.

Clinicians have necessarily to work within such limitations, while being prepared to advocate for greater flexibility in what can be prescribed. A further difficulty in some countries is regulations that enforce stringent procedures for the prescription of opioids. Individual practitioners may be required to obtain a special licence before they may prescribe the drugs, special forms will need to be completed for each prescription, and regular reports completed on opioid use.

Starting an opioid

Having determined that pain is not controlled by adequate doses of non-opioid medications such as NSAIDs, or weak opioids such as tramadol or dextropropoxyphene, it is time to introduce a major analgesic, an opioid.

Since an effective dose can be determined only by trial, it is usually recommended that treatment starts with low doses of short-acting formulations administered as frequently as necessary to control pain, increasing successive doses at regular intervals until satisfactory pain control is attained.

A common approach would be to prescribe the following (see Tables 11.7.1 and 11.7.2):

- *morphine solution 5 mg/ml susp.* 5–10 mg by mouth 3–6 hourly allowing the patient or those administering the drug to gauge the most useful dose and time interval of administration within those limits.

An alternative might be:

- *oxycodone 5 mg tab.* 1–2 tab. every 3–6 h or
- *hydromorphone 1 mg/ml susp.* 1–2 mg every 3–6 h;
- methadone equivalents cannot be given with any confidence, because of the variable half-life, which leads to accumulation of the drug in some individuals.

Table 11.7.1   *Useful preparations of opioids*

Drug	Formulation	Dose range/use
Morphine		
	1, 2, 5, 10 mg/ml susp.	Oral dose is approximately
	5, 10, 20, 30, 50, 60, 100, 200 mg CR tab.	three times the injected
	5, 10, 15, 30 mg (sulphate) inj.	dose; and up to 20 times
	120 mg (tartrate)	the epidural dose
Hydromorphone		
	1 mg/ml susp.	No dose range
	2, 4, 8 mg tab.	CR formulations are
	2, 10 mg/ml inj.	in some countries available
Oxycodone		
	5, 10, 20 mg immediate release tab.	Ampoules for injection are
	10, 20, 40, 80 mg CR tab.	available in some countries
Methadone		
	10 mg tab.	Long half-life, which is also
	10 mg/ml inj.	very variable
	5 mg/ml solution	
Diamorphine		
	5, 10, 30, 100, 500 mg inj.	Available in UK, commonly
		used in syringe-drivers
Fentanyl		
	Trans-dermal patch,	Re-apply each 2–3 days; reserve
	2.5, 5, 7.5, 10 mg	for baseline analgesia

CR: controlled-release formulation.

Table 11.7.2   *Approximate equivalent doses of common opioids*

	Oral	Parenteral	Epidural
Morphine	10 mg	3–5 mg	0.25–1.0 mg
Oxycodone	5 mg	4–5 mg	–
Hydromorphone	1.5–2 mg	1.0–1.5 mg	0.1–0.4 mg
Methadone	*	*	–
Fentanyl	–	50–100 μg	5–20 μg
Diamorphine	–	2–4 mg	
Codeine	60–120 mg	–	–

*No clear equivalent for methadone; its variable and prolonged half-life can cause accumulation at quite low doses.

Conversion from one opioid to another cannot be precise; there is great variation between individuals. Therefore, when changing opioids, start the new drug at the lowest end of the suggested range of equivalence, and be prepared to increase the dose depending on the response of the patient.

Some simple rules provide useful guidance
- The dose of injected morphine (subcutaneous (S/C) or intravenous (I-V)) is approximately one-third of the oral dose.
- Oral oxycodone doses are approximately one-half the equivalent dose of oral morphine.
- Hydromorphone oral dose is approximately one-seventh the equivalent morphine dose.
- The dose of injected fentanyl (measured in micrograms) is approximately one-hundredth the equivalent oral morphine dose.

Baseline and break-through (rescue) analgesic doses

Once a regular dose that controls pain is established, a controlled-release formulation can be started, its dose calculated by adding up the total dose required through 24 h, and prescribing that amount in two divided doses at 12-h intervals. This gives a continuous, baseline level of analgesia.

Fentanyl is a popular alternative opioid in many places where there is a common fear of morphine because of its perceived addiction potential or a view that it accelerates the progress of disease. But fentanyl is not a useful drug to start with, being available in most centres only as a transdermal patch with the smallest one delivering 600 μg over 24 h, equivalent to approximately 50 mg of oral morphine, and that may be an excessive dose for an opioid-naïve person.

However, once satisfactory control of pain is achieved with immediate release preparations, if the total 24-h dose required is more than 50 mg morphine or its equivalent, a 25 μg/h fentanyl patch may be very appropriate therapy.

As pain is most commonly variable, in addition to a continuing baseline form of analgesia, there must be break-through (or rescue) doses ordered, to be taken as necessary for 'break-through' pain in the period between the times baseline drugs are administered. Usually the break-through dose will be approximately one-sixth of the total daily dose being administered as baseline. It may be the same opioid as the baseline medication or a different preparation. (If a fentanyl patch is used for baseline, break-through usually will be given as morphine, hydromorphone or oxycodone, if the oral route is possible.) In non-malignant disease break-through pain has been described as common, frequent, short lasting and unpredictable. Sometimes it is 'incident pain', related to movement or posture.

Side-effects of opioids

Patients and carers should be warned about the common side-effects of an opioid:

Drowsiness. If this is an isolated difficulty, not a component of overwhelming fatigue, the use of methylphenidate is often helpful:

- *methylphenidate 10 mg tab.* 10 mg in the morning, repeated if necessary at midday.

Nausea. Common when first starting an opioid, this side-effect may resolve after a time. Occasionally it is persistent and very troublesome, and requires a change to a different opioid. It is usual to offer, alongside an opioid, a prescription for an antinausea medication that can be taken regularly before meals as necessary:

- *metoclopramide 10 mg tab.* 10 mg tds;
- *domperidone 10 mg tab.* 10 mg tds.

Confusion and delirium. Any opioid may cause delirium, and this may be subtle ('I just don't feel right in myself') or frank confusion with hallucinations and bizarre behaviour. There seems to be an unpredictable individual variation in opioid receptor profiles at the neuronal level that determines that one opioid will be better tolerated than another. If morphine causes hallucinations, for example, these may disappear after a change to oxycodone or fentanyl; if confusion follows administration of fentanyl, it may be worth suggesting a change to an equivalent dose of hydromorphone. In either case it may be appropriate to reduce the dose or change to another opioid, and if this is not practicable, the use of psychotropic medication may control most of the difficulty:

- *haloperidol 0.5 , 1.5, 5 mg tab.* 0.5–5 mg bd.

Constipation. The effect of virtually any opioid in reducing bowel activity is such as to make it mandatory to order aperient medication in conjunction with an opioid:

- *docusate 50 mg + senna 8 mg tab.* two tablets at night, any day bowels not open.

Myoclonus. In some individuals, opioids cause intermittent jerking movements of muscle groups. The causative dose varies widely, some persons being much more susceptible to this complication than others.

If the symptom is troublesome, use antispasmodic medication, for example:

- *clonazepam 1 mg tab.* 0.5–1 mg bd.

NEUROPATHIC PAIN

Recognition and assessment

Neuropathic pain is recognized by one or more of four basic characteristics:

1. There is pathology present (or presumed) that has potential to damage nerve cells or nerve fibres.
2. There is change in or loss of sensation or reduced muscle power in that part of the body served by the potentially damaged nervous tissue.
3. The character of the pain experienced is described as of a burning or pins and needles quality, or comes with sudden shooting jabs.
4. There is a relatively poor response to common analgesics such as paracetamol or opioids.

Clinical examination will include a careful search for evidence of neurological defect in the region of the pain sensation, and in particular areas demonstrating allodynia, hyperalgesia, dysaesthesia, mapping their limits for comparison with later examinations, usually with the aid of a body diagram.

Management

There is not a single management strategy that will be appropriate for all neuropathic pain. It is commonly necessary to experiment with a number of therapies before finding one that suits an individual patient best. Research in this area has commonly been confined to management of diabetic neuropathy or localized neuropathic pain – post-herpetic or trigeminal neuralgia, and the pain presentations seen in degenerative neurological conditions are often more complex. The analgesics used for nociceptive pain (especially opioids) still have an important part to play, and should be increased as necessary, to whatever dose level is effective and avoids side-effects. Different opioids have different receptor profiles; oxycodone, for example, may target the κ (kappa) receptor, whereas morphine and fentanyl have their action primarily at the μ (mu) receptor. Both oxycodone and tramadol appear to have a better effect on neuropathic pain than morphine, and methadone also is considered helpful for difficult pain when used in addition to another opioid, even in relatively low dose: 10–20 mg bd.

Membrane stabilizers

The adjuvant drugs that will be more predictably useful in many cases of neuropathic pain are the membrane stabilizers. 'Membrane stabilizer' is a useful but non-specific term to describe their presumed mechanism of action. To explain the mechanism of action of a drug to patients is difficult when our own knowledge of the mechanism by which it acts is quite limited. However the following approach is generally helpful. As in epilepsy, where one can envisage nerve cells firing off excessively and that excess being stopped by anticonvulsants, in neuropathic pain we can envisage an abnormal and increased excitation of neurones and excess transmission of impulses in nerve fibres subserving pain. That increase is reversed by anticonvulsants. Antidepressants, similarly, act to reduce the 'noise' in the nervous system that makes depressed persons sleepless and agitated; antidysrhythmics reduce the intensity of the nerve impulses stimulating cardiac muscle.

These very simple concepts are undoubtedly quite inadequate, even incorrect, as explanations of how these drugs work. It is likely that at least some anticonvulsants block sodium channels, but others may act through an effect on gamma amino butyric acid (GABA) receptors. As is not unusual in therapeutics, we use these drugs because they work, not because we understand precisely their mechanisms of action.

It is important to individualize doses for the use of all these classes of medications, and some common principles need stressing:

- Most are taken by mouth, and oral absorption may vary considerably.
- Some agents are bound to plasma proteins and are affected by protein levels and the co-administration of other drugs.
- Some are cleared by the liver, others excreted by the kidney; effective action of these drugs may therefore be affected by hepatic or renal disease.
- All have side-effects: common ones are somnolence, dizziness; and sometimes skin rashes can be quite severe.

Which drug?

Individual variation makes it difficult to determine which drug to introduce as a first choice. For lancinating, shooting, sudden pains, most clinicians will start with an anticonvulsant; for burning pain, with an antidepressant. But often it will be necessary to combine both classes of drugs, along with an opioid. Some prefer old and trusted medications, others look to the supposed advantages of newer drugs. Medications for neuropathic pain are commenced at a low dose and the response is reviewed daily for effectiveness and undesirable side-effects. As necessary, doses are increased every 2 or 3 days, usually to a recognized maximum level.

Anticonvulsants
- *carbamazepine 100, 200 mg tab.; 200, 400 SR tab.* 100 mg bd, increasing to 400 mg bd or more;
- *sodium valproate 100, 200, 500 mg tab.; 200 mg/5 ml susp.* 100 mg bd increasing to 600 mg bd or more;
- *sodium phenytoin 30, 100 mg tab.; 100, 250 mg I-V inj.* 300 mg daily increasing to 600 mg daily or more;
- *gabapentin 300, 400 mg cap.; 800 mg tab.* 300 mg daily or bd, increasing to 600 mg tds or more;
- *clonazepam 0.5, 2 mg tab.* 1 mg bd increasing to 2 mg bd or more;
- *lamotrigine 2, 5, 25, 50, 100 mg tab.* 50 mg daily increasing to 200 mg bd or more.

Antidepressants
- *amitriptyline 10, 25, 75 mg tab.* 25 mg daily, increasing to 150 mg daily.

Other tricyclic antidepressants in similar doses.

- *paroxetine 20 mg tab.* 20 mg daily increasing to 60 mg daily.

Newer SSRI antidepressants do not seem to be as effective as the tricyclics.

Antidysrhythmics
- *mexilitine 50, 200 mg cap.* 50 mg tds increasing to 200 mg tds or more;
- *flecainide 50, 100 mg tab.; 10 mg/ml inj.* 50 mg bd, increasing to 200 mg bd or more;
- *lidocaine (Lignocaine) 20 g/ml, 100 mg/ml* by S/C infusion 1–2 g over 24 h;
- *lidocaine 5% patch* (up to three patches applied to the area of maximal pain for no more than 12 h); titration is unnecessary.

OPIOIDS IN CHRONIC PAIN

The use of opioid analgesics commonly has been limited to the relief of acute severe pain or of cancer pain, because of the fear of addiction or abuse. The prolonged use of opioids in chronic pain is achieving greater recognition as an appropriate strategy, but some simple rules apply.

Continuing use of an opioid will often lead to tolerance (requiring higher doses of opioid to achieve analgesia). This is rarely a problem, and doses can be increased as necessary.

Tolerance may be accompanied by dependence, meaning that withdrawal of the opioid will lead to uncomfortable symptoms – restlessness, sweating. Again this is rarely a cause of difficulty if the withdrawal is done progressively over a period of days or weeks.

The risk of addiction (a craving for the opioid) is unusual when treatment has been initiated for major pain, and will be minimized if only *controlled-release formulations* are employed to avoid peaks and troughs in opioid blood levels that may initiate withdrawal symptoms and foster addictive behaviour.

Opioid use over a prolonged period sometimes promotes a paradoxical effect, an abnormal pain sensitivity with hyperalgesia. Apart from the perceived risk of inducing addiction behaviour, this phenomenon has reinforced the need for caution in introducing opioid therapy for non-cancer chronic pain. It is recommended that management be undertaken by a single physician who is able to ensure that, if non-opioid treatment has failed, a continuing therapeutic relationship with the patient can be established to ensure comprehensive monitoring and effective follow-up.

CENTRAL PAIN

Central pain occurs in a number of circumstances. It is most easily understood when it arises following a stroke. Neuronal damage gives rise to discomfort some time later, often a month or more following the stroke, and this may confuse the diagnosis. Central pain may cause severe distress, but be vague in its description and difficult to localize, and may change over time. Somatosensory disturbances may accompany central pain, and damage to spinothalamic tracts is suggested as a facilitating factor in its initiation. Depression, anxiety and sleep disturbances commonly occur. Amitriptyline is recommended as the first line of treatment; other antidepressants, anticonvulsants and opioids may also prove beneficial, as used in neuropathic pain. Oral or parenteral ketamine has been effective in some cases (p. 109).

Peripheral nerve injury has also been suggested as a contributor to the development of central pain, through central sensitization affecting dorsal root ganglion cells in the spinal cord, with the *N*-methyl-D-aspartate (NMDA) receptors in the dorsal horn assuming a major significance. Anatomic changes in dorsal root ganglia and dorsal horn cells include sympathetic nerve sprouting and a risk of sympathetically maintained pain and regional pain syndromes. Once these anatomical changes have occurred, central pain may continue even after the cessation of an initiating pain stimulus – sometimes called *autonomous pain*. Treatment is often unrewarding; there should be a search for any remediable stimulus factors such as an operable neuroma or treatable neuropathy, with an attempt to reduce any inflammatory component at a site of injury with NSAIDs, and the use of tricyclic antidepressants, anticonvulsants or S/C or I-V lignocaine infusion (which may acutely reduce discomforts of hyperalgesia and allodynia).

Sympathetic blockade is undertaken for regional pain syndromes and reflex sympathetic dystrophy, and dorsal column stimulation or intrathecal delivery of morphine, clonidine or ketamine may be suggested. These are best supervised by a specialist pain clinic.

OTHER STRATEGIES FOR DIFFICULT PAIN

Local opioids for pressure ulcer pain

Pain due to pressure ulcers does not respond well to oral analgesics. Some success has been reported with the use of topical opioid gels, the opioid solution mixed into a stable sterile gel by the local pharmacy.

Ketamine

Ketamine is an NMDA receptor antagonist, and has proved useful in situations of desperate pain, which will often have a neuropathic or central component. It may be administered by mouth, but is commonly given as a S/C or I-V infusion, starting with 25 mg as a trial bolus, and if well tolerated and showing some effect, going on with a 24 h infusion of 100–400 mg plus rescue bolus doses of 25–50 mg 2–4 hourly as necessary:

- *ketamine 200 mg/2 ml inj.* In a continuous S/C or I-V infusion it is compatible with many other medications (e.g. morphine, fentanyl, metoclopramide, haloperidol, midazolam).

Some patients experience hallucinations on ketamine and require the addition of a benzodiazepine (midazolam).

Epidural and intrathecal drugs

For mixed or neuropathic pain in the lower extremity, the delivery of medication via an indwelling epidural or intrathecal catheter accessed through a S/C portal can be very effective. The catheter will usually be placed in position in a pain management unit, and an initial programme of drug administration by this route advised by staff of that unit. Morphine is given epidurally in much lower doses (one-tenth to one-twentieth of the daily S/C dose) and also less frequently (8–12 hourly). If morphine by mouth or by injection or infusion is causing persistent nausea, if doses are escalating to very high levels, if confusion is limiting the doses that can be used, a change to epidural administration might be considered. It can be combined with local anaesthetic, which diminishes the transmission in spinal fibres. Fentanyl and hydromorphone can also be administered by the epidural or intrathecal route:

- *morphine 10 mg/ml inj.* 1–20 ml bd–tds;
- *bupivicaine 0.25–0.5% 2–10 ml bd–tds;*
- *fentanyl 100 μg/2 ml inj.* 25–200 μg bd–tds;
- *hydromorphone 1 mg/ml, 10 mg/1.5 ml* 1 – 10 mg bd–tds.

These drugs can also be administered in a continuous infusion feeding into the S/C portal, but this increases the risk of introducing infection to the epidural space.

In addition, adjuvant medications have been shown to have effect by this route, either by bolus injections two or three times in 24 h, or added to a continuous infusion. They include:

- *clonidine 150 μg inj.* 50–100 μg;
- *ketamine 100 mg/ml inj.* 10–50 mg;
- *midazolam 5 mg/ml inj.* 2.5–10 mg.

As is commonly the case in managing chronic pain, the effectiveness of any intervention for difficult pain cannot be predicted with any confidence; it is important to monitor the effect carefully, and be prepared to regard each prescription as a trial, ready subsequently to maintain, reduce, increase or abandon it.

8

Cognitive, behavioural and psychological symptoms

COGNITIVE IMPAIRMENT

Global cognitive impairment, such as is seen in dementia, embraces learning, memory, motor skills and social skills. Selective loss of only some of these functions also occurs, and may be potentially reversible, being caused by anxiety, personality change or organic depression. Some degree of cognitive impairment is a feature of Parkinson's disease, Huntington's disease, progressive supranuclear palsy, cerebral tumour and the late stages of multiple sclerosis (MS).

Causes of cognitive impairment that are partially or completely reversible include hypoxaemia, hypercalcaemia, renal failure, hepatic failure, urinary or respiratory infection, hypothyroidism, B12/folate deficiency and depression. Medications that can cause cognitive impairment include benzodiazepines, opioids, tricyclic antidepressants (TCAs) and drugs with anticholinergic activity. There may be a pre-existing or emerging psychiatric disorder.

The challenge for the neurologist is to distinguish reversible conditions from those requiring only symptomatic treatment. Even in advanced disease, potentially reversible causes will usually be treated. It may be impossible to cease all potentially causative medications without a return of unacceptable symptoms (e.g. pain) but substitution of one drug by another may give significant improvement, for example substitution of oxycodone or fentanyl for morphine may reduce confusion or hallucinations.

Cognitive impairment may be subtle and unrecognized by family members, who may interpret changes in behaviour as indicating emotion or anger. They will be grateful for support in devising simple strategies to help compensate for impairment in the patient. Memory difficulties may be assisted by simple routines such as the use of lists or the display of written reminders. In MS, cholinesterase inhibitors, corticosteroids or interferons may bring about a time of improvement, and the use of rivastigmine may improve memory for a time.

DELIRIUM, AGITATION AND RESTLESSNESS

Delirium is a disturbance in consciousness, cognition and perception. It may be a brief episode, be intermittent in occurrence or extend over a prolonged period. Its basic characteristics are a failure of attention, and impaired levels of consciousness and consequent impairment of cognitive function. There may be agitation and hallucinations. Delirium needs to be distinguished from dementia and from psychosis, and an underlying cause should be sought, because it may be readily reversible.

The supportive phase
There are a number of tools devised for the diagnosis of delirium; but a useful bedside test is a simple question 'Do you feel clear in the head?' or 'Do you feel confused?' Some patients will recognize that their hallucinations are unreal, or will confess that they do not feel quite clear.

The search for cause will include consideration of recent changes in drug administration or withdrawal, infection, hypoxia, metabolic changes and dehydration.

Any potential cause should be corrected if possible. If, for example, delirium is due to an opioid or steroid drug, a change in analgesic or withdrawal of the steroid may effect an improvement.

While considering causes, it will be important to seek immediate relief of the discomfort of agitation and confusion; a cause of distress to the patient, bewilderment to the family and an unwanted demand on staff.

Non-pharmacological interventions can be very useful, such as structuring the environment so that it promotes a calm and supportive ambience. Simply leaving a light on, encouraging a sleep routine, providing the continuing presence of a family member or friend or volunteer, ensuring adequate fluid intake, allowing some movement out of bed and removal of restraints (e.g. intravenous (I-V) line or catheter) can all assist. Education for family and caregivers may be necessary to help them create and maintain that helpful environment, and maintain routines and safety.

Oral medications to relieve agitation and confusion:

- *haloperidol 0.5, 1.5 mg tab.* 0.5–5 mg bd-tds depending on response;
- *diazepam 2, 5, 10 mg tab.; 10 mg inj.* 10–20 mg orally as a single dose, this may be repeated every 2–6 h, up to 120 mg daily, depending on the response.

- *chlorpromazine 10, 25, 100 mg tab.; 5 mg/ml susp.; 50 mg inj.* 50–100 mg (tab. or susp.) orally, repeated every 2 h, up to a maximum of 300 mg in 24 h;
- *thioridazine 10, 25, 100 mg tab.; 10 mg/ml susp.* 50–100 mg (tab. or susp.) orally, repeated every 2 h, up to a maximum of 300 mg in 24 h.

Chlorpromazine and thioridazine may cause postural hypotension. If high doses are found necessary, the patient should be nursed in bed.

Alternative medications are:

- *olanzapine 2.5, 5, 7.5, 10 mg tab.; 5, 10 mg wafer.* 10–20 mg/day as a single dose; its availability in a wafer formulation that disperses in the mouth can be an advantage.

Other alternatives include risperidone, pericyazine, lorazepam and promethazine.

Parenteral medications

- *haloperidol 5, 10 mg inj.* 5–10 mg S/C (up to a maximum of 30 mg in 24 h), dose may be repeated in 15–30 min, if required;
- *midazolam 5, 15 mg inj.* 2.5–5 mg subcutaneously (S/C), as a single dose (monitoring patients for excessive sedation, respiratory depression or hypotension);
- *diazepam 10 mg inj.* 5–20 mg I-V, as a single dose, titrated to response; this should be given by slow I-V injection over several minutes to minimize the risk of respiratory depression or arrest;
- *droperidol 2.5, 10 mg inj.* 2.5–10 mg S/C (up to a maximum of 30 mg in 24 h), dose may be repeated in 15–30 min, if required;
- *zuclopenthixol acetate 50 mg inj.* 50–150 mg S/C, as a single dose (not to be repeated for 2–3 days).

Flumazenil 0.5 mg inj. 0.2 mg up to 1 mg I-V will reverse acute benzodiazepine sedation.

Haloperidol is the first choice. The dose will vary greatly, some individuals becoming calm and responsive with doses of only 1 mg; others requiring up to 30 mg in 1 day, so repeated administration of small doses is appropriate, titrating up to what produces the desired effect. An important advantage of haloperidol is its suitability for administration by S/C injection or continuous infusion.

Extrapyramidal side-effects or hallucinations may be sufficiently severe to require withdrawal of the drug. If tardive dyskinesia occurs it may be necessary to administer benztropine 1–2 mg, repeated as necessary.

Haloperidol is not consistently sedating, and if sedation seems advantageous, midazolam may be added, and is compatible in the same syringe, 2.5–5 mg as a bolus, 5–15 mg by continuous infusion over 24 h.

In severe cases of distressing agitation propofol in a dose of up to 10 mg/h can be administered, preferably via a central line.

The terminal phase: 'terminal restlessness'

This is a term given to a form of agitated delirium which may present in the last days or hours of life. It is characterized commonly as 'picking at the bedclothes'. Restless movement and repetitive vocalization suggests distress for the patient, and is upsetting for watching family, inhibiting any opportunity for communication. If the symptom accompanies marked deterioration, and is of fairly recent and sudden onset, the search for cause may be inappropriate, but more often it will be a phase in the progressive decline of a dying person.

A choice then presents itself – provide increased sedation to help the patient be less restless (which will make the possibility of further exchange with the patient unlikely), or withhold that sedation in the hope that the patient will remain aware of the surroundings and remain able to communicate in some way. Some observers will regard sedation as accelerating the approach of death, yet the situation may be distressing for family, as well as, perhaps, for the patient. Family can be asked to assist in the decision as to whether to withhold sedation as an attempt to maintain contact, or administer it in the knowledge that death is imminent anyway and that any possible distress can thereby be hopefully palliated:

- *midazolam 5, 15 mg inj.* 10–30 mg S/C infusion/24 h, together with analgesics, etc.

DEPRESSION

Psychological problems are common in neurological patients but may be insufficiently recognized or considered in planning programmes of care. In traumatic brain injury, stroke, Parkinson's disease, MS, epilepsy and brain tumours affective symptoms can accompany impairment in brain functioning and be important contributors to morbidity. Because the neurological disorders themselves may cause cognitive and emotional deficits, the presentation of depression in these patients can be complicated.

The association of depression with loss, and the many losses that are part of the progression of a chronic neurological disease (loss of work, loss of mobility, loss of speech, loss of independence of many kinds) should bring to consideration the question of whether depression is contributing to patient distress in such conditions.

Psychopharmacological treatments are appropriate in the treatment of depression in patients with neurological illness, but patients with both depression and a neurological illness may not respond to conventional anti-depressant treatment as well as those with major depression alone.

In depression following stroke, these medications are regarded as safe and effective:

- *citalopram 20 mg tab.* up to 60 mg/day;
- *sertraline 50, 100 mg tab.* up to 200 mg/day;
- *fluoxetine 20 mg tab.* up to 80 mg/day.

In dementia, also, some efficacy has been claimed for these medications.

In Parkinson's disease some effect has been claimed for agents that can block re-uptake of dopamine (e.g. tricyclic antidepressants TCAs). However, tremor, seizures, akathisia, myoclonus, dyskinesia and delirium have been described as side-effects of TCAs in neurological patients.

ANXIETY

Anxiety accompanies many stressful life situations and it might be expected to occur in progressive neurological diseases such as amyotrophic lateral sclerosis (ALS) or Parkinson's disease.

Expressions of anxiety may point to underlying disturbances of depression, delirium, pain, isolation or fear. Simple companionship, explanation and opportunity to ventilate fears and expectations may be sufficient to allow patients to cope with their anxiety.

If pharmacological assistance proves necessary, benzodiazepines will assist both mood and sleep. Commonly used formulations are:

- *temazepam 10 mg tab.; 10, 20 mg cap.;*
- *oxazepam 15, 30 mg tab.;*
- *lorazepam 1, 2.5 mg tab.;*
- *alprazolam 0.5, 1 mg tab. 0.25–0.5 mg.*

Occasionally in elderly persons, these agents cause excitement rather than sedation:

- *haloperidol 1.5, 5 mg tab.; 5 mg inj.* may be more effective, particularly if there is agitation and some confusion.

In advanced and terminal disease, midazolam, clonazepam and haloperidol may all be administered by subcutaneous injection either as repeated bolus doses or as a continuous S/C infusion.

INSOMNIA

Management of sleep difficulty is not simply a matter of finding a better sedative. First explore what can be done to establish a more effective and comfortable sleep routine without the use of medication. Avoid daytime naps, stop any use of alcohol or caffeine, set regular times for sleep and being awake, or, for patients with normal cognitive ability, introduce a simple relaxation routine.

Difficulty in sleeping is commonly considered under three headings:

Difficulty in getting to sleep.
Frequent waking through the night.
Early morning wakefulness.

Persons who have difficulty getting to sleep may have a higher level of arousal at the time of going to bed, caused by any of a wide variety of influences: some personal – pain, anxiety, despair, upset following an argument; some environmental – noise, light, lack of privacy, strangeness of surroundings, unfamiliar bed. A significant number (up to 30% in older age groups) will be affected by periodic limb movement or restless legs (pp. 60–61).

Some who wake often through the night are not troubled by their wakings. They may need to pass urine, or wake for only a short time and return promptly to sleep again; others remain awake for long periods, the mind 'busy' with unwelcome thoughts, and unable to 'switch off'. An important subgroup will have snoring or sleep-apnea problems causing repeated episodes of hypoxia. Others will have evidence of depression.

Those who wake early share some of the characteristics of the second group. They may also have been using sedatives with a relatively short half-life, and wake after the effect of the drug has worn off.

In each group some common potential disturbances may prevent a good sleep, and may be amenable to change: indigestion and bowel upsets, muscle aches and cramps, joint pains, urinary urgency, shortness of breath and orthopnoea, cough, changed temperature regulation, nightmares, fear of falling out of bed, drugs that alter usual sleep patterns. The chronic use of sedatives may inhibit sound sleep; other drugs that affect sleep adversely include steroids, anticonvulsants, anti-Parkinson's drugs, opioids, selective serotonin reuptake inhibitors (SSRI) antidepressants and anticholinergics. Many of these contributors to a poor sleep are found in patients with neurological diseases.

For those who have trouble getting to sleep, a benzodiazepine will usually initiate sleep in the short term. Prolonged use risks dependence and a lack of effect:

- *temazepam 10 mg tab.; 10, 20 mg cap.*

The clinician should avoid, if possible, simply adding sedatives, but from an assessment of the type of ineffective sleep, choose either a single appropriate agent or a combination of several. If muscle or joint pain or skin ulceration is a cause of discomfort in bed, a simple analgesic:

- *paracetamol 0,5 g tab.; cap.* 1 g repeated 4–6 hourly or
- *morphine 10 mg tab.; 1, 2, 5 mg/ml susp.* 5–10 mg may be most useful.

If anxiety or restless legs cause arousal:

- *clonazepam 0.5, 2 mg tab.* or
- *carbidopa–levodopa (25 mg carbidopa + 100, 250 mg levodopa)* may be more effective.

If there is frequent wakening through the night because of urinary urgency, the addition of baclofen and reduction in evening fluid intake may assist, and a small dose of TCA will smooth out a pattern of repeated wakeful periods, and allow the patient to 'switch off' the mind and return to sleep easily:

- *Amitriptyline 10, 25, 75 mg tab.* 10–25 mg early in the evening.

If sleep apnoea and hypoxia is involved (e.g. especially in ALS) consideration may need to be given to the use of assisted ventilation with BiPAP (pp. 72–73).

Patients with dementia may demonstrate the phenomenon of 'sundowning', being wakeful and restless in the late afternoon and evening, and also confused, aggressive and disorientated.

Melatonin 2 mg tab. has been claimed to calm some and help induce sleep; others may respond better to dopamine antagonists:

- *clozapine 25, 100 mg tab.* 12.5–25 mg or
- *risperidone 1, 2, 3, 4 mg tab.* 1–2 mg or
- *olanzapine 2.5, 5, 7.5, 10 mg tab.; 5, 10 mg wafer.* 1–15 mg.

These compounds are also useful in the psychosis that can accompany Parkinson's disease.

GRIEF AND BEREAVEMENT

The acceptance within palliative care of an interest in and responsibility for family members as well as individual patients, has led to a common extension of care into the bereavement period, seeking to assist family members cope with their grief. This represents a quality of care that deserves to be included within the remit of neurologists. Many patients with neurological diseases die after long illnesses during which the neurologist has provided the major professional support. During this time there will often have been numerous consultations with family members, and if they have felt a close relationship with their neurologist during that time, they will appreciate an occasional contact after death has occurred.

Bereavement is a state of loss, a time when adjustment to the absence of an important 'other' is necessary. Grief is the emotional response of those who have suffered the loss and is a common human experience, one that may become a very difficult and complex matter in some circumstances. Mourning is expression of that grief, influenced by many personal, historical and cultural factors.

There are a number of recognized factors that can give warning of complicated and difficult grief. Sudden unanticipated death, suicide, death of a child, change in circumstances as a result of the death, previous experiences of loss or lack of available family supports may all lead to a very distressing or prolonged bereavement period.

In such circumstances grief can be profound and intense, with development of depressive or anxiety disorders and poor physical health.

There is a common pattern to the way grief is experienced over time following a loss, and sometimes it will be possible to discern the well-known stages of numbness, yearning, despair and reorganization that were described by Kubler–Ross. Those classical 'stages' are by no means usual, and sometimes there is a delay in the onset of grief. Follow-up over quite a long period may be necessary if support is to be useful.

Suggested tasks for the grieving person include acceptance of the reality and finality of the loss, facing and expressing the pain of grief, adjusting personal life to the fact that the person has indeed gone, and reappraising the significance of the lost relationship and moving into a new pattern of life. Bereavement support groups provide safe settings where feelings of loss can be readily expressed without any expectation of 'moving on' and appear to be welcomed by those whose grief is uncomplicated, and who may not have actually needed any special intervention.

For complicated grief, there is little evidence that any particular therapy is effective in relieving and facilitating a satisfactory bereavement. But it is important to try to identify those persons at risk of a complicated grief, and be able to suggest a referral option by which they can be offered individual counsel and support.

It will not be necessary for the neurologist to become trained as a grief counsellor, but in accepting in clinical practice a palliative approach to the care of advanced and terminal neurological illness, it will be appropriate to know something of normal and abnormal grief, and, following the death of a long-term patient, to be aware of the resources that can be made available to families who have long relied on neurology advice and care.

9

Miscellaneous symptoms

TEMPERATURE CONTROL AND PYREXIA

Fever is a complex physiological response triggered by infectious or septic stimuli. Elevations in body temperature occur when concentrations of prostaglandin E(2) (PGE(2)) increase within certain areas of the brain. These elevations alter the firing rate of neurons that control thermoregulation in the hypothalamus. Although fever benefits the non-specific immune response to invading microorganisms, it is also viewed as a source of discomfort and is commonly suppressed with antipyretic medication.

Antipyretics such as aspirin work by inhibiting the enzyme cyclooxygenase and reducing the levels of PGE(2) within the hypothalamus. They may also reduce pro-inflammatory mediators, enhance anti-inflammatory signals at sites of injury, or boost antipyretic messages within the brain.

In polyneuropathy (e.g. type 2 diabetes mellitus), the ability of skin blood vessels to dilate is impaired. This impaired vasodilatation leads to an increased risk of heat illness during exposure to elevated ambient temperatures.

Ageing alters physiological responses to cold stress and heat stress, and responses alter further, depending on fitness level and the effects of chronic disease that may change the normal mechanisms of peripheral vaso-constriction, cold-induced metabolic heat production, sweating and cardiovascular function.

SWEATING (HYPERHIDROSIS)

More than one-half of patients with Parkinson's disease complain of sweating disturbances that are not correlated with disease severity, but do match other symptoms of autonomic dysfunction. They report physical, social and emotional impairments due to sweating that relate mainly to autonomic dysfunction, 'off periods' and dyskinesia.

Severe hyperhidrosis can cause extreme embarrassment that may lead to social and professional isolation. Treatment options differ in their invasiveness and efficacy and include antiperspirants, iontophoresis, cholinergic inhibitor drugs, botulinum toxin and surgical sympathectomy. Particularly in advanced and terminal conditions, the least invasive treatment that provides effective symptom control should be sought, because evidence to support one treatment over another is lacking.

Medications have won a place for the relief of sweating in palliative care patients, but none is consistently effective for all patients. They include:

- *cimetidine 400 mg bd;*
- *thioridazine 10 mg nocte;*
- *benztropine 0.5 mg tds;*
- *propantheline 7.5–15 mg tds;*
- *venlafaxine 37.5–75 mg once or twice daily.*

Sympathetic blockade: medical (clonidine, prazosin or phenoxybenzamine) or by sympathetic block using phenol may also be employed.

Intradermal injections of type A botulinum toxin reduce excessive sweating when it is more localized (e.g. palmar hyperhidrosis in a fixed clenched fist).

PRURITIS

There are many causes of symptomatic pruritis (itch), but few relate directly to neurological disorders. Along with xerosis (dry skin), pruritis is the most common dermatological problem for the aged residents of chronic care facilities, leading to stasis dermatitis and ulcer formation. The maintenance of an adequate ambient humidity is helpful, and setting out a basin of water lessens the drying effect of air conditioning. Cooling the skin relieves pruritus by directly inhibiting cutaneous sensory receptors.

Among a variety of local applications to relieve pruritis, moisturizers are key components. Creams, which are oil-in-water preparations, are more hydrating than lotions, which are usually powder in water. Ointments are the most hydrating; they contain petrolatum and are occlusive, minimizing evaporative losses.

Topical applications include:

- *menthol and camphor in combination;*
- *pramoxine hydrochloride, a topical anaesthetic used alone or with hydrocortisone;*

- *capsaicin 0.025%, 0.075% cream for itchy psoriasis;*
- *doxepin hydrochloride 5% cream.*

Drug therapy should be initiated in severe or persistent itch. Low-sedating antihistamines have a place in therapy but are non-specific:

- *doxepin 10, 25 mg cap.; 50.75 mg tab.*, a tricyclic antidepressant, is a potent systemic H_1-histamine receptor antagonist;
- *cholestyramine 4, 8 g powder pack*, a basic anion exchange resin which is not absorbed from the gastrointestinal tract lowers the serum bile acid concentration in patients with cholestasis and may also assist uraemic pruritus.

Other medications effective in cholestatic pruritis include opioid antagonists (*naloxone*) and *rifampicin 150 mg bd.*

HICCUPS

Hiccup is an intense synchronous contraction of the diaphragm and intercostal muscles lasting about 0.5 s and followed by glottal closure, which gives it a characteristic sound. Common causes of hiccups are of gastrointestinal origin, with gastric distension or other pathology causing local irritation of the diaphragm or disturbance of the vagus nerve, but they may also be caused by diseases in the medulla – infarction, tumour or infection – or complicate metabolic derangements such as uraemia.

Some drugs – alcohol, opioids, steroids and sedatives have been claimed to occasionally induce the symptom.

Although most attacks of hiccups cease spontaneously, persistent discomfort can be extremely distressing and have a significant impact on quality of life. Simple non-pharmacological interventions that activate the vagus nerve may be effective, including naso-pharyngeal stimulation (e.g. sipping iced water or provoking a sneeze), sucking on a strong peppermint sweet, compressing the eyeballs or re-breathing from a paper bag.

Hiccups caused by brainstem pathology or metabolic disorders will usually require pharmacological measures:

- *chlorpromazine 10, 25, 100 mg tab.* 25–100 mg has been commonly employed;
- *baclofen 10, 25 mg tab.* 10–30 mg tds is now usually preferred.

Other drugs recommended include:

- *metoclopramide 10 mg tab.* 10–20 mg tds;
- *nifedipine 10 mg tab.* 10 mg tds.

Valproic acid, cisapride, omeprazole and gabapentin have also been reported as effective.

There are numerous folklore remedies claimed to relieve this symptom, and many reports of acupuncture proving effective. Other heroic measures include phrenic nerve block, vagal stimulation and sphenopalatine ganglion block.

HEADACHE

In family practice, tension headache and migraine are common diagnoses for individuals presenting with headache. Persons with late stage neurological conditions may experience the same range of headaches.

Other possible diagnoses include:

- post-traumatic headache after cranial injury;
- headache from cerebral tumour;
- morning headache due to hypoxia;
- headache associated with depression;
- headache due to degenerative cervical spine disease;
- neuralgia in the area of the face and head.

When the patient is elderly, the headaches that are more common in old age need consideration:

- temporal arteritis;
- temporo-mandibular joint disease;
- post-herpetic neuralgia;
- Paget's disease.

Symptomatic management may require frequent use of analgesics – paracetamol or an opioid either as required or on a regular basis, but other specific interventions may be more appropriate for particular conditions:

- Ventilation support for hypoxic headache.
- Injection of trigger points or use of acupuncture in myofascial disease.
- Non-steroidal anti-inflammatory drugs (NSAIDs) for degenerative spinal disease.

- Corticosteroids for temporal arteritis or cerebral tumour.
- Antidepressant medication.
- Dental opinion on temporo-mandibular dysfunction.
- Local capsaicin cream, and wrapping the affected area with cling film to protect it against local stimulus in post-herpetic neuralgia.
- Membrane stabilizer drugs for neuropathic pain – tricyclic antidepressants or anticonvulsants (p. 106).

SECTION III

Major Neurological Conditions Requiring Palliation

1

Cerebrovascular disease: stroke

Stroke is usually a dramatic event; unlike the progressive neurological deterioration of amyotrophic lateral sclerosis (ALS) or Parkinson's disease, and its outcome is difficult to predict. The sudden onset of stroke may call for urgent interventions to reduce progression or extension of brain damage, including administration of aspirin, thrombolytic drugs and blood pressure reduction, plus supportive care – intravenous (I-V) hydration, investigation of cause, prevention of deep vein thrombosis (DVT), early mobilization and appropriate diet. From that acute presentation approximately one third will die within days, one third will achieve a complete or partial recovery, and one third will not improve, and risk further deterioration and eventual death. That last group will be left with severe brain damage, be at risk of severe disability and major discomforts; it is for them that palliative management is most appropriate.

SUPPORTIVE PHASE

The initial symptoms and discomforts common in stroke will be treated expectantly, looking for improvement and encouraging an emphasis on rehabilitation. Where there is further deterioration, emphasis shifts to the maintenance of comfort. There are common difficulties for these patients requiring careful analysis and specific interventions if quality of life is to be satisfactory.

Palliation issues
Bulbar symptoms, swallowing and communication difficulties
Bulbar symptoms may occur through paralysis of motor speech functions, specific damage to cerebral speech areas and connections, or more complex psychological effects with restlessness and anxiety compromising

self-awareness and impairing patient descriptions of discomfort. Difficulty in communication means that patients are unable to verbalize clearly and are at risk of being misunderstood and having their needs not adequately met. Locked-in syndrome is a special and frightening case, and its recognition may be missed (p. 212).

Maintenance of nutrition and hydration

Loss of ability to swallow effectively is a threatening symptom triggering great anxiety and fear of choking. Nutrition and hydration are both compromised, requiring decisions about whether nutritional and hydration support via feeding tubes is appropriate; these decisions may present great difficulty for both staff and family members.

Immobility, pressure ulcers

Immobility causes frustration and despair, can lead to fixation of joints, with stiffness and pain apparent on movement, and cause painful pressure areas and breakdown of skin. Home management will be assisted by the availability of appropriate equipment (inflatable mattress, electric bed, lifter, wheelchair, etc. – see Practical aspects for home care in Chapter 1 of Section V, p. 225).

Pain

Pain in paralysed muscles and immobile joints or arising from pressure ulcers is largely nociceptive in type, and benefits from regular analgesia (the World Health Organization (WHO) ladder) but also from regular passive movement, massage and measures to prevent contractures (see Management of nociceptive pain in Chapter 7 of Section II, p. 100; Muscle spasm, pp. 50–53).

Central pain – a neuropathic-type pain presumed due to nerve damage, particularly in the area of the thalamus, corpus striatum and parietal lobe – may be difficult to express and localize, and may vary over time. Sometimes pain may be felt in the area of the body corresponding to the involved portion of the cerebral hemisphere (see Neuropathic pain in Chapter 7 of Section II, p. 105). Antidepressant medications usually have a better effect than carbamazepine.

Psychological symptoms: confusion, depression

Confusion and restlessness, an abnormal sleep pattern, panic attacks, and persistent anxiety may occur after a stroke, and require quite large doses of benzodiazepines or neuroleptics to achieve acceptable calm (see Confusion and delirium in Chapter 7 of Section II, p. 104).

Depression is commonly associated with loss, and the losses that accompany a severe stroke are manifold: loss of ability to self-care, to move, to speak, to feed, to think clearly. In some studies, but not all, tricyclic antidepressants have been demonstrated to be useful, as have more selective serotonin uptake inhibitors (e.g. citalopram, fluoxetine).

Cognitive impairment will cause difficulty for care by family members. Recurring small strokes or transient ischaemic attacks (TIAs) are a cause of dementia, and more specific cognitive disabilities in sensory appreciation, thought processes or ability to express needs, call for patience and persistence on the part of those who provide support.

Bladder and bowel disturbances

Incontinence of urine is a common problem, and an embarrassment to the aware patient. The presence of a urinary tract infection should be checked and treated appropriately. Where prognosis is judged to be poor, a condom drainage device or an indwelling catheter will usually be welcomed. Careful protection of skin from pressure effects will be particularly important where there is either urinary of faecal incontinence. Immobility leads to constipation that needs always to be kept in mind as a potential cause of faecal incontinence (see Constipation in Chapter 5 of Section II, p. 82).

Venous thrombosis

In the weeks following a stroke, patients are prone to venous thrombosis and consequent risks of leg oedema and pain, and pulmonary embolus. Where there are factors favouring recovery from stroke (young age, early indications of reduction in paresis, etc.), it may be appropriate to start a preventive regimen for DVT with daily low-molecular-weight heparin (enoxaparin) injections 1 mg/kg body weight.

Chest infection

Inability to move, or to cough effectively and clear pharyngeal and bronchial secretions inevitably makes a patient prone to chest infection, indicated by fever, more rapid breathing and cough. Antibiotic treatment may prove effective; sometimes it will be an appropriate decision (made with patient or relatives) not to treat such an infection (which in former days was often called 'the old man's friend' – a comfortable final stage of illness).

Mortality and quality of life

Death following a stroke results primarily from neurological complications in the first month. Up to 80% of persons afflicted by a severe stroke maybe expected to die within 6 months, often from a chest infection or cardiac cause (dysrhythmias, myocardial infarction). Although major discomforts following a severe stroke may seem to have left a victim in a very unfortunate state, many individuals who suffer a persistent hemiplegia and aphasia indicate that their quality of life is acceptable to them.

THE TERMINAL PHASE

Palliation issues
Site of care
Either because of shortage of bed places or because funding arrangements give preference to cancer and human immunodeficiency virus (HIV) patients for hospice-type care, admission to a specialized unit for terminal care (e.g. a hospice) will rarely be available for victims of stroke. There is no doubt that the high staff–patient ratios and the excellent preparation of staff for care of dying persons that characterize the best hospice units are entirely appropriate for the terminal care of severe stroke, but nowhere in the world is there ready availability of such facilities for stroke patients. What will improve the care for those who have poor recovery and progressive deterioration after stroke is a full appreciation within stroke units, neurology wards and aged care facilities of the palliative management approach, and a willingness, where opportunity allows, to engage with and liaise with palliative care expertise.

Management of discomfort: pain, restlessness, confusion
As with any advanced disease where mobility is very impaired, simple movement for hygiene purposes or skin protection may provoke pain, evinced by groaning or grimacing. Regular doses of analgesia and sedation, administered by mouth or tube feeding or (often preferable) by the subcutaneous (S/C) route – intermittent or as a continuous infusion is a compassionate contribution to care, and is much appreciated by family members:

• *morphine 10–15 mg + midazolam 5–10 mg or clonazepam 1 mg over 24 h.*

Nutritional support, initiation and withdrawal of tube feeding
Nutrition presents a major dilemma. Inability to swallow sufficiently well to maintain body weight is a poor prognostic sign. The naso-gastric feeding tube has been a common mechanism for introducing liquid feeds, but is uncomfortable and demeaning; per-endoscopic gastrostomy (PEG) feeding

is now more available, but, as with naso-gastric feeding does not improve survival markedly. Where the patient is judged to be unconscious, repeated discussion with family members may be necessary about whether to continue feeding at all, and if so, by what method.

If the patient is perceived to suffer thirst, regular ice chips by mouth and frequent mouth care may assist comfort, or a continuous S/C infusion of 1 l of fluid (saline or dextrose/saline) over 24 h is usually tolerated on a continuous basis; but whether it alters prognosis is doubtful.

2

Demyelinating disease

Multiple sclerosis (MS) is the most common condition in this group of diseases. It is characterized by two distinct pathological processes: the development of inflammatory plaques throughout the central nervous system and progressive axonal degeneration. It is usually regarded as an autoimmune disorder, stemming from a combination of unknown environmental factors and genetic predisposition.

It is a disease that affects mainly younger adults; it has a variable course, often there are periods of relapse and improvement, but overall a progressive deterioration, which may occasionally be rapid, but more usually is prolonged, extending even for decades (Figure iii.2.i). The prolonged natural history of the disease means that it is rare for one physician to follow an affected person throughout its entire course.

Not all cases will follow a steadily progressive intermittent course. Three main forms are recognized:

1. relapsing and remitting MS (illustrated);
2. primary progressive MS in which remissions do not occur;
3. secondary progressive disease where progression occurs late in the disease.

Diagnosis and prognosis

Magnetic resonance imaging (MRI), along with cerebrospinal fluid (CSF) analysis, has made it more possible to be definite about the diagnosis in the early stages. As initially the long-term outlook cannot be predicted with any certainty, the way in which the disease and its potential discomforts are discussed at the time of diagnosis assumes major importance. There are some agreed indicators that may be helpful in guiding predictions of a favourable or unfavourable prognosis. An older age of onset, multiple symptoms at onset, pyramidal and cerebellar symptoms and a short interval between relapses all indicate more rapidly progressive disease.

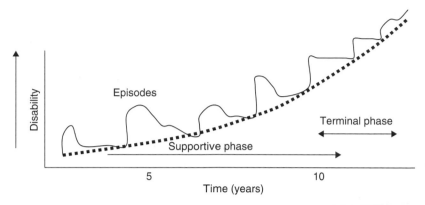

Figure III.2.1 The recurrent relapses characteristic of MS and the progressive but variable increase in disability.

The extent to which a realistic appraisal of the future is shared with the patient and family will be guided by both individual and cultural considerations. Denial is a defence mechanism that may need to be respected; truthful responses to direct questions are usually appropriate, but should be judged with compassion and sensitivity in the amount of detail necessary. Within the families and community groups that provide support for MS sufferers there is an abiding interest in new research aimed at clarifying the basis for myelin damage in MS and determining how it might be delayed or reversed. It is a field of science that is changing rapidly, and it will be natural for hope to be maintained in the expectation of some scientific 'breakthrough' promising effective treatment. Such advances remain elusive, and for any individual, the frustrations of continuing deterioration may be compounded by a fear that any new findings will come too late to be useful.

SUPPORTIVE PHASE

Palliation issues

Prognosis uncertainty

The future outlook for a person with MS is uncertain. As a rough guide, 30% of affected persons do well, and maintain an active life; 10% do badly and experience progressive decline. Approximately 60% will continue a meaningful life for years, but be subject to unpredictable relapses and slowly deteriorating function in several or most areas of life. Initially, the major issues for patients and families are psychological rather than physical, relating to the uncertain future of the disease and its potential consequences for the ability to work and to earn a living. The approach of caring professionals should be positive and encouraging focused on maintaining function and preserving well-being. Where necessary, advocacy at the usual place of employment for the patient to continue a normal round of daily activity may be appropriate. Later, a recommendation of reduced hours or modification of tasks to suit better an impaired physical status may be helpful.

Management of relapses

Relapses commonly include exacerbations of local and general weakness, visual loss, incontinence, fatigue and depression. Acute relapses have commonly been treated with a pulse of corticosteroids given over 3–4 days:

- *methylprednisolone 0.5, 1.0 g inj.* 1 g/day; or
- *dexamethasone 8 mg inj.* 16 mg/day, which speeds the return of function, but does not improve the degree of subsequent recovery.

When, during relapses, new symptoms arise, they should be met with consistent encouragement, accompanied by specific palliation approaches.

In more affluent countries medications designed to delay relapses and modify progress of the disease are commonly used. Interferon beta, for example, having an immune-modulatory function, can delay relapses when given early in the course of the illness, and has become standard therapy where it can be made available. Side-effects (flu-like symptoms, injection-site reactions or depression) may abort this treatment; further, it is very expensive and may fail to demonstrate any appreciable benefit, which can cause the patient additional disappointment. An alternative is daily injection of *glatiramer acetate* 20 mg, the structure of which resembles that of myelin, and which appears to downregulate immune responses.

In people with worsening or progressive disease, mitoxantrone reduces relapses and slows progression. However, it is associated with a dose-related cardiomyopathy and can cause leukopenia and other side-effects. Very preliminary findings of the effect of *simvastatin* 80 mg daily over 6 months suggest a cautious hope of improvement in the clinical deterioration and the number of gadolinium-enhancing lesions on MRI brain scanning.

Importance of teamwork

The wide range of disorders possible in MS calls for the deployment of many skills. If these are to be managed optimally, an integrated, cooperative approach by a team that includes professionals from the mix of physician, physiotherapist, speech therapist, occupational therapist, psychologist, social worker and nurse will be necessary. Such a team may not be immediately apparent, and may need to be found, recruited and gathered around the patient's needs. In situations where such resource persons may be unavailable the primary physician will need to have some practical understanding of how to initiate simple useful interventions that encourage maintenance of function. It will often be family members who are best placed to give continuing support, and ways of underpinning their interest and augmenting their skills can be crucial. The unpredictable timing of relapses, some occurring no more frequently than once per year, highlights the desirability that team support be available at all times, even though continuing supervision may seem unnecessary to many patients.

Information and support

If there are locally available lay support groups for MS they will often be a major resource; providing information about equipment and respite opportunities, carer education, specialist services and current research on drug therapies. Many patients and their family carers will undertake detailed research in libraries or web sites, bringing a considerable knowledge to their consultations, but perhaps also at risk of diversion into unproven and alternative treatments, sometimes highly expensive.

Use of alternative medicine

Among chronic neurological diseases MS is one in which patient and family members very commonly seek the assistance of alternative practitioners. Its unpredictable and irregular course, characterized by relapses and improvements offer a fruitful field for unconventional interventions that, given lucky timing, may claim that a particular technique has been responsible for improvement. Some families may readily be exploited by unscrupulous practitioners (see Working alongside complementary and alternative medicine in Chapter 5 of Section I, p. 40).

Common symptoms

MS affects diverse areas of function, causing motor and sensory disturbances, cognitive impairment, mood disorders, psychosis, sphincter problems, fatigue and reduced mobility. The symptoms most commonly met with are bladder dysfunction, fatigue, spasticity, neurobehavioural complaints and mood disorders, pain syndromes, tremor and ataxia. Many are frequently under-treated.

Bladder dysfunction. It is a major cause of distress and embarrassment and is almost invariable. Urinary symptoms may be primarily irritative, obstructive or both. Urgency, frequency, incontinence and bladder spasms or hesitancy causing retention are common problems (see chapter Urological

Symptoms in Section II, p. 89). Improved control may result from monitoring fluid intake in advance of times when opportunity to pass urine is restricted; other non-drug treatments include pelvic floor training and the use of biofeedback techniques.

Medications can reduce painful spasms: for example, oxybutin, propantheline, hyoscine (but these may induce retention). Frequency may be reduced by tricyclic antidepressants. Nasal desmopressin is sometimes useful. Self-catheterization is practised successfully by some patients, but for others a better solution may be permanent drainage via a supra-pubic drain rather than a urinary catheter. Electrical stimulation of an implanted bladder stimulator is sometimes undertaken, or of the hypogastric plexus to encourage voiding by stimulation of sympathetic nerves.

Fatigue. This is experienced in up to 90% of MS patients. It will often be worse after any activity, after a hot bath or in a hot environment and be helped by cooling drinks, cool baths and environment, and summer clothing. Maintaining regular exercise within the limits enforced by weakness will usually be helpful.

Antidepressant medication may help:

- *fluoxetine 20 mg cap.* 20–40 mg;
- *sertraline 50 mg tab.* 25–100 mg daily.

Some success is reported for the following:

- *amantadine 100 mg cap.* 100 mg bd–tds;
- *modafinil 100 mg tab.* 200–400 mg daily either as a single morning dose or divided twice a day may have a better effect;
- *methylphenidate 10 mg tab.* 10 mg a.m. and midday may reduce the sleepiness which accompanies fatigue (see chapter Fatigue in Section II, p. 45).

Impairments of movement. Loss of power and impairment of coordination contribute to impaired mobility and frustration. Loss of vision and difficulty in speech inhibit communication. Physiotherapy (stretching exercises, massage and encouraging effective use of functioning muscle groups) can do little to speed recovery from a relapse, but it can lessen consequent disability by encouraging better use of what function remains and provide useful emotional support even if a measurable improvement in physical capacity is not attained.

Similarly, coordination difficulties are approached by introducing the use of mobility aids that can offer improved control. Much will depend on available resources, social supports and the individual's cognitive function, mood and motivation.

Flexor spasms with muscle pain are an outcome of spasticity, and further reduce movement. A number of antispasmodic drugs are useful, including baclofen and dantrolene. Baclofen can also be used intrathecally (see p. 53). Affected muscles may go on to fixed contractures and deformities that are painful and cause considerable difficulties for daily care.

Tremor and ataxia occur with cerebellar involvement. Treatment is often unsatisfactory, but a number of medications are commonly prescribed (p. 60). Weighted bangles, worn on the wrists, help control movement for feeding or when undertaking hand crafts.

Swallowing difficulties may result from impairment of ability to chew and of reflex coordination of the passage of food into and down the oesophagus. Speech therapy expertise may assist a greater awareness of the swallowing action; also teaching best posture for times of swallowing, and active exercises for relevant muscles. Modification of the diet (thickened fluids or vitamised solids) will need individual assessment.

Pain and sensory disturbances. In MS, pain may be of several types:

- acute paroxysmal neurogenic pain from ectopic excitation at sites of demyelination as occurs in trigeminal or glossopharyngeal neuralgia;
- subacute pain from bladder spasm, or pressure sores;
- musculoskeletal pain from strained muscles, inactivity, spasms, restless legs;
- chronic pain from dysaesthesia in the extremities, or spasm of muscles.

There may be burning pain, paraesthesiae and sudden shooting discomfort in the limbs or across the trunk. Episodes are unpredictable, occurring spontaneously and often last only a brief time. There is a temptation to treat sudden severe pain with injectable opioid which has a fast effect, but blood levels also decline quickly and there is a risk of inducing psychological dependence, even addiction. If opioids are to be used, the more persistent background pains of muscle ache and joint stiffness are a better target, using long-acting medications such as transdermal fentanyl or sustained-release morphine if non-steroidal anti-inflammatory drugs (NSAIDs) are ineffective or cause side-effects.

Anticonvulsant drugs (carbamazepine, valproate) are often preferred for paroxysmal neuropathic pain; tricyclic antidepressants (amitriptyline, imipramine) for persistent burning discomfort. Antidysrhythmics (mexilitine, infusions of lignocaine) or baclofen or clonazepam should also be considered. No one agent will be useful for all patients (see Neuropathic pain in Chapter 7 of Section II, p. 105). For painful bladder spasms oxybutynin 5–10 mg bd is recommended (p. 91).

Paroxysmal phenomena may recur in MS, but seizures are uncommon. Paraesthesiae, clumsiness, speech difficulty, double vision, weakness or vertigo can occur spontaneously; and as for paroxysmal pain may be reduced by the same anticonvulsants suggested for neuropathic pain.

Episodes of sudden visual loss from optic neuritis usually recover spontaneously.

Musculoskeletal pain responds best to applications of heat, massage, stretching exercises and NSAIDs.

Chronic neurogenic pain usually responds best to tricyclic antidepressants and similar drugs, for example:

- *amitriptyline 10, 25, 75 mg tab.* 10–75 mg early in the evening;
- *capsaicin 0.025%, 0.075% cream* (increasing to the stronger preparation if tolerated) applied to the painful area tds is a useful adjunct;
- *clonidine 100, 150 µg tab.* 150–300 µg tds may be added.

Any discomfort, including pain, is likely to be experienced more intensely when there is also depression, isolation and a lack of activity or distraction. Sometimes a clinician will judge that a discomfort is being 'exaggerated'. An intimate and compassionate response may find ways to give at least some relief through better understanding of the emotional context of the discomfort, without either ignoring the patient's distress or prescribing.

Bowel dysfunction. Constipation in up to one half of patients occurs through reduction in fluid intake, immobility and drugs with anticholinergic effect. If constipation is so severe as to cause unrecognized faecal impaction causing spurious diarrhoea with anal leakage, it risks being inappropriately treated with antidiarrhoeal agents, increasing the problem.

Psychosocial issues

The diagnosis of MS is difficult to accept, and denial is a common response, sometimes leading to rejection of medical help, and search for alternative 'cures' (pp. 40–41). Affective disorder is very likely to occur and there is an increased risk of suicide. Selective serotinin reuptake inhibitor (SSRI) antidepressants may be helpful, or lithium if there is a bipolar component.

The diagnosis of MS has a major effect on family life, and appropriate and acceptable social arrangements for care are of great importance. Many patients are relatively young, married and with young families. Marriage breakdown is not unusual, especially if the patient is the female partner. There are likely to be problems with employment and finance, the matter of retaining a driving licence, and issues of the custody and care of children. The many disturbances of function that occur in MS inhibit socialization, and reduce opportunity for exchange and the formation of friendships. Changes in emotional expression and impairment of cognitive ability interfere with relationships.

Within established partnerships, sexual drive may remain but failure of erection in males and ability to orgasm in females limits satisfaction. The use of sildenafil and related medications (tadalafil, vardenafil) has been suggested for its potential to benefit sexual performance and response in males. The efficacy in females is much less certain.

Site of care

Many health services will have difficulty in locating a suitable placement for a severely disabled, relatively young person with advanced MS. Opportunity for short-term respite placement to allow caring family members a time of relief from the burden of care can be most helpful. A specialized hospice unit will not usually accept such a patient because of an uncertain length of prognosis and limited bed numbers. 'Nursing home' placement is usually reserved for the elderly; acute hospital placement is seen as unnecessary, expensive and inappropriate. Each population area of around one half to one million persons will benefit from the availability of special in-patient unit(s) established to accommodate young persons damaged by degenerative neurological disease, cerebral trauma or severe cerebral palsy. Otherwise these unfortunate patients may be directed to peripheral or marginal in-patient settings where little expertise relevant to their care is available.

THE TERMINAL PHASE

Palliation issues

Motor impairments: weakness, wasting, contractures

The final stages of MS are often characterized by established contractures, immobility, extreme fatigue, gross wasting and weakness. The permanence of functional defects becomes more and more evident. The ability to perform even the simplest movements is increasingly impaired, and there is complete dependence in a world that is increasingly limited to one uncomfortable posture, in one bed or chair, in one room. Communication fails; pain medications, antispasmodics and sedatives further cloud intellectual ability. Carers experience recurrent despair and some may begin to hope that the patient will find a quick release from what sometimes seems a prolonged torture.

Cognitive impairment: memory loss, poor concentration

Deterioration in short-term memory occurs, with slowing and poor organization of thought, and difficulty in concentration and decision-making.

Psychological changes: lability of mood, depression

Lability of mood, with outbursts of laughing or crying (a pseudo-bulbar effect) may occur and respond to one of the SSRIs, for example:

- *citalopram 20 mg tab.* 10–60 mg/day.

Loss of vision increases feelings of frustration, fear and total dependency.

Skin care

In the later stages pressure ulcers are a major risk through immobility, restricted choice of posture, loss of sensation, incontinence and poor nutrition. Meticulous attention to cleanliness, and care in regular re-positioning is essential, and the use of air mattresses and cushions to localized skin pressure can be most helpful.

Bowel management

Shame and embarrassment is caused by bowel accidents, and training to encourage the bowel in a regular evacuation should be undertaken, with attention to fluid intake and the regular use of aperients, suppositories or enemas.

Administration of medications

Continuous infusion of medications, such as opioids, lignocaine, clonazepam and baclofen may be the best way to ensure some measure of patient comfort. Hydration may become difficult to sustain, and a per-endoscopic gastrostomy (PEG) may need consideration if swallowing is severely impaired and thirst a problem. A subcutaneous litre of saline or dextrose/saline over 24 h can also be tried as a short-term measure.

Management of terminal events

The cause of death in MS is commonly respiratory (pneumonia, aspiration pneumonia, pulmonary embolus) or renal (renal failure, urinary infection).

Falls resulting in hip fracture may occur, and pulmonary emboli follow deep vein thrombosis related to inactivity. In one study, death from suicide was over seven times more common in MS patients than in a control group. Suicide may be sought more often by individuals feeling a lack of strong personal supports. Infection is the major common terminal event that might be treated, but whether it requires treatment is something to discuss, if possible, prior to its onset.

Advance directives

If it can be predicted that a patient faces a prolonged, variable but often progressively downhill course, the writing of an advance directive would seem to be a useful preparation. It could guide decision-making towards the end, when poor cognitive function may preclude full patient participation. But individuals with MS often die from an acute unanticipated event, and the struggle to maintain dignity and function through so many times of relapse and partial recovery fosters, for many, a confidence in being able to carry on. It will be very difficult to anticipate future outcomes or prepare guiding directions (see chapter Advance Directives in Section IV, pp. 205–206). Without such guidance, however, it can be difficult for close family members to make irreversible decisions about treatment when a patient has lost the capacity to form and express an independent opinion.

This is also a circumstance that arouses interest in physician-assisted suicide. This remains an intervention forbidden by law throughout the world except in one or two countries. A more widely countenanced option is to refrain from active treatment of (for example) respiratory infection, or other intervening conditions that seem likely to end life (see chapter Euthanasia in Section IV, p. 219).

3

Parkinson's disease and related disorders

There are a number of degenerative syndromes less common than Parkinson's disease in which parkinsonism (the triad of rigidity, tremor and bradykinesia) occurs and for which care requires similar considerations. Each of these conditions may have a particular emphasis in its mix of symptoms. Patients with multiple system atrophy (MSA), for example, are more likely to have troublesome urinary incontinence compared with Parkinson's disease patients and MSA more often causes early erectile dysfunction. Other syndromes include progressive supranuclear palsy (PSP), dementia with Lewy bodies (DLB), corticobasal degeneration (characterized by asymmetric parkinsonism) and Parkinson's disease with dementia (PDD). These conditions do not, on the whole, respond to therapy as well as does Parkinson's disease, and their 'atypical' nature may become clearer through a lack of response to levodopa (L-dopa).

The principal clinical feature of Parkinson's disease is bradykinesis, slowness of muscle contraction, along with muscle rigidity and tremor (mainly at rest). Muscle stiffness results in slowness of movement. Patients are forced to adopt a stooped posture, and proceed with shuffling short steps. There is imbalance and patients are prone to falls. The face is impassive, body movement may be suddenly frozen. Constipation and urinary symptoms more typical of prostatism occur.

THE SUPPORTIVE PHASE

The course of Parkinson's disease is commonly described as one of up to 5 years with acceptable control of symptoms, then increasing disability and difficulty for another 5 or more years. With older patients, the length of these periods may be considerably shorter, and some will die before the disease expresses itself fully.

Younger individuals may remain independent for up to 15 years, and initially have no need for specific medication. At some stage, however, difficulties that limit function in unacceptable ways will require drug therapy. Older individuals with Parkinson's disease are prone to acute co-morbidities such as trauma due to falls and vascular disorders that may precipitate social problems. Multi-disciplinary networks covering regional community settings are useful in assisting both the clinical and social problems that are encountered.

Palliation issues

Motor dysfunctions

Motor dysfunctions include tremor, muscle rigidity, instability, fear of falling, speech. Muscle rigidity and slowing of contraction lead to a lack of confidence in undertaking more complex physical activities, and of performing simultaneous or sequential tasks. Daily activities, such as eating a meal, getting dressed or going to the toilet may become major difficulties. Individuals most at risk of frequent falls are those with more severe disease who show a marked response to L-dopa treatment, and have more dyskinesia and 'on–off' phenomena. Fear of falling contributes to postural instability, depression and anxiety. Regular physical therapy improves balance and confidence.

Resting tremor may be mild, or quite disabling and a major embarrassment. Where it is the major manifestation of the disease, in younger patients, anticholinergic drugs and dopamine agonists are the mainstays of treatment, but side-effects limit their use in older persons (see Tremor in Chapter 2 of Section II, p. 59).

Difficulty in speech, in swallowing, in turning in bed, in writing and in dressing reduce independence and erode personal dignity. A marked slowing of all activity requires great patience on the part of carers.

Constipation is a common problem, as is nocturia, urgency and urinary frequency.

Autonomic dysfunctions: postural hypotension, abnormal sweating, erectile failure

Autonomic dysfunctions include:

• Orthostatic hypotension, which increases the risk of falls, and may force reduction in L-dopa and other drugs. It can be sufficiently severe to require increased salt intake or fludrocortisone.

- Increased sweating results from impaired thermo-regulation, and may respond to beta-blockers.
- Erectile dysfunction (pp. 93–94).

Cognitive impairment and psychological difficulties

Cognitive impairment, hallucinations, agitation, depression, anxiety and panic attacks may all complicate the illness and increase the difficulties for both patients and carers.

Sleep disturbance, nightmares and restless legs syndrome trouble the night hours.

Drug therapy

From the broad spectrum of possible symptoms, one patient may experience a particular selection; another patient may be afflicted by a quite different selection.

The aim of treatment is to keep affected individuals mobile, independent and socially active for as long as possible, and that this is attempted by prescribing a range of medications. The physical manifestations of the disease respond best to the L-dopa range of drugs:

- *carbidopa-levodopa (25 mg carbidopa + 100, 250 mg levodopa)*, a variable dose regimen depending on individual response.

This will frequently be used in combination with a dopamine receptor antagonist, for example:

- *bromocriptine 2.5 mg tab.; 5 mg cap.* 2.5–7.5 mg bd;
- *cabergoline 0.5 mg tab.* 0.5–2 mg bd;
- *pergolide 50, 250 μg tab.* 50–750 μg bd.

These agents are the mainstay of supportive care during the long period of slowly progressive deterioration. Their effect may 'wear off' in time, requiring increased doses, while peak dose effects may cause involuntary movements, and there is a risk of precipitating psychosis in elderly persons. Benzhexol and benztropine have a role in the control of salivation and painful dystonia, but can exacerbate mental deterioration and are less often used.

Non-drug therapies

These continue to be important to patient and family. A clear understanding of the nature and the natural history of Parkinson's disease is a necessary basis for recruiting family members as effective carers, helping them to become patient and sympathetic supporters of the patient's daily living, and to access appropriate equipment and nursing support for home care. The support of a multi-disciplinary team can prove invaluable, with useful input from physiotherapist, speech therapist, occupational therapist, dietitian and social worker. Community groups and organizations that gather patients and caring families for education and mutual support, build awareness and confidence in care.

THE PHASE OF TRANSITION

The change from supportive to terminal phase will often be difficult to mark with any clarity. Much will depend upon the cognitive capacity of the patient, and how clearly individual wishes are able to be formulated and expressed. As symptoms become more obvious and distressing in spite of large doses of L-dopa, attention naturally shifts to other symptom control measures.

Palliation issues
Place of neurosurgical intervention
Treatments for Parkinson's disease tend to be effective early in the disease, and discomfort may be controlled for decades with drug therapy and/or neurosurgical interventions (deep brain stimulation). Criteria for under-taking deep brain stimulation are becoming more firmly established as well as characteristics of the clinical course that rule it out (e.g. atypical parkin-sonism, dementia, other brain pathology, poor social support).

Cognitive and psychological impairment, hallucinations
Greater cognitive and psychological disturbances commonly supervene in the later stages of the disease, and complicate the physical disability, with both depression and pain as frequent symptoms. If care is being supervised by a family physician, it may be helpful to seek specialist neurological advice. Carers also find these later symptoms much more difficult to cope with than physical disability. Hallucinations may accompany cognitive decline, and increase with higher doses of L-dopa. Cholinergic drugs may give some temporary improvement. Cholinesterase inhibitors may improve cognition:

- *rivastigmine 1.5, 3, 4, 5, 6 mg cap.* 1.5–6 mg bd.;
- *donepezil 5 mg tab.* 5–10 mg/day.

Psychotic episodes may require the use of the neuroleptic clozapine (an occasional cause of agranulocytosis):

- *clozapine 25, 100 mg tab.* 12.5–400 mg/day.

Psychiatric symptoms (as with other forms of dementia) are common precipitants of re-admission for institutional care.

If hallucinations are a major concern, L-dopa may need to be reduced or ceased. Faced with a choice of being either stiff and immobile or hyperactive, some patients will elect to employ their drugs to focus on a short period of activity each day – a little segment of acceptable life – rather than risk a daily succession of highs and lows.

Motor impairment: dyskinesia, speech and swallowing difficulties

Management of motor impairments remains essentially palliative. Bulbar and pseudo-bulbar lesions cause difficulty in speech and swallowing, dysphagia and the risk of aspiration and chest infection (see Dysphagia in Chapter 3 of Section II, p. 65). Dyskinesia leads to physical exhaustion and compounds weight loss from poor nutrition. Sleep is often disturbed by physical and mental restlessness and repeated dreaming, and may be relieved by:

- *clonazepam 0.5, 2 mg tab.; 1 mg inj.* 0.5–2 mg at night.

Protection against damage caused by bumping into domestic objects may be achieved by the use of hip pads.

Communication problems

Communication becomes more difficult, and non-verbal cues are difficult to read in the mask-like facies.

Bladder and bowel dysfunction

Bladder dysfunction may require an indwelling catheter or supra-pubic drainage. Care must be taken to avoid constipation and faecal impaction, requiring regular attention with osmotic softeners or enemas.

Skin care

Skin care may be compromised by seborrhoeic dermatitis – a further feature of the spectrum of Parkinson's disease.

THE TERMINAL PHASE

It is in the final stages of the prolonged course of Parkinson's disease that discussion with patient and family will seek agreement that the focus of management will shift from maintenance of maximal function to best degree of comfort.

Palliation issues

Medications

The commonly used dopaminergic drugs and antidepressants are available only by mouth, and up to the terminal phase, every effort has been made to continue them. Now, even controlled-release formulations of these drugs become more and more difficult to administer comfortably, and may be better stopped. Loss of control makes the patient prone to fall, and reduction of medication and use of a wheelchair may be better accepted now. Continuous infusions of apomorphine may be employed when oral medication can no longer be swallowed:

- *apomorphine 10 mg/ml inj.* 50 mg over 24 h.

This is a time also to assess the value of other oral medications that may exacerbate confusion (sedatives, anticholinergics), or lower blood pressure or increase bulk in stools.

Sleep difficulty

Sleep is made difficult by limitation in the postures that can be maintained by stiff limbs (which may now also have established contractures) and a stiff trunk, and may be further impaired by restless legs and limb pain.

Skin care

Airflow mattresses help the skin, but the patient will still need to be gently repositioned regularly to maintain limb comfort. Meticulous attention to the skin will be necessary to avoid pressure sores.

Sedation and analgesia

In the final stages of the disease, techniques commonly employed include a continuous subcutaneous (S/C) infusion of opioid, anti-emetic (domperidone) and sedation:

- *clonazepam, 0.5, 2 mg tab.; 1 mg inj.* 0.5–1 mg given twice daily by S/C bolus or as a continuous infusion (2 mg/24 h);
- *morphine 5, 10, 15 mg inj.; midazolam 5, 15 mg inj.* Morphine 10–30 mg + midazolam 5–10 mg over 24 h by infusion may moderate hyperkinesis and emotional distress.

Avoid haloperidol in Parkinson's disease.

An advance directive will be helpful if it confirms the physician's judgement to focus on comfort as a primary aim, and authorizes rejection of measures such as intravenous hydration or antibiotic treatment of chest infection when these are regarded as inappropriate, or unlikely to be effective.

4

Dementia

Dementia is the term used for a number of conditions in which there is intellectual deterioration accompanied by a progressive decline in independence and a shortened life expectancy. Alzheimer's disease is the most frequent diagnostic label; it indicates a primary disorder of neurones and a characteristic neuropathology. There are a number of other causes of dementia, including fronto-temporal and Lewy body types. Cerebrovascular disease is a common additional cause.

Old age is the strongest risk factor for dementia, and it has been estimated that its prevalence in the USA in person over 80 years of age exceeds 20%. The increasing proportion of elderly persons in virtually all populations indicates a progressive and global rise in the burden of care for demented persons.

The focus of this discussion will be on Alzheimer's disease, in which four stages may be recognized in its evolution and progress, though these are rarely clearly defined:

1. *An early stage* when mild cognitive impairment limits ability to perform routine complex tasks such as cooking, but allows self-care in matters of personal hygiene.
2. *A moderate stage* in which the individual is able to walk without help, but needs assistance to undertake basic activities of daily living, and requires oversight to prevent unsafe activity.
3. *A severe stage* in which the individual is unable to walk without help or self-feed, but there is preservation of basic communication.
4. *A final stage* with inability to walk even with assistance, or to communicate in any meaningful way.

Major dilemmas for the exercise of care in dementia arise in stages 3 and 4, when assessment of discomfort is made difficult by the patient's inability to report symptoms with any clarity or to indicate the effectiveness of treatments designed to maintain comfort.

SYMPTOM MANAGEMENT IN DEMENTIA

A central aim for care in dementia is the maintenance of comfort, dignity and quality of life. Interventions to maintain comfort will not necessarily be pharmacological; rather they will often require psychosocial and environmental considerations.

In a society that values wit and quickness of thought, it is easy for individuals with dementia to be devalued, marginalized and reduced to their disease ('only a case of dementia').

Palliation issues
Appropriate medications
Medications are used to treat cognitive and non-cognitive symptoms. Acetylcholinesterase inhibitors are commonly used to assist cognitive function, though their beneficial effect is often slight. They include:

- *donepezil 5 mg tab.* 5–10 mg/day;
- *rivastigmine 1.5, 3, 4, 5, 6 mg cap.* 1.5–6 mg bd;
- *galantamine 4 mg tab.* 4–8 mg/day.

Non-cognitive symptoms include delusions, hallucinations, sleep disturbance, agitation, depression, anxiety, apathy, disinhibition and aberrant motor behaviour.

Family support
Family support should receive emphasis through the long course of dementia, whether through offering respite opportunities or by the availability of support groups where carers may ventilate feelings of frustration or guilt.

Home care will often provide the most satisfactory environment for the patient, being quite familiar and offering known consistent carers. There are heart-warming accounts of spouses who have consistently provided skilled and loving attention to help the patient live as fully as possible and retain some sense of self. However, home caregivers also commonly report that they feel 'on duty' 24 h a day. Most will have needed to give up employment. Particularly in the patient's final phase of life carers commonly experience depressive symptoms. Respite opportunities for family relief are a necessary component of community dementia care.

Symptom recognition, including pain

Symptom assessment should be global rather than focused on any particular feature. In an individual who cannot communicate effectively, there may still be observable signs or behaviours by which to differentiate one symptom from another among the possible causes of discomfort.

In institutional settings, consistent staff will come to know their patients' patterns of behaviour and be ready to recognize deviations that could indicate discomfort. They will be helped by a tool such as a simple clinical checklist which gives vocabulary for reporting the recognition of distress, and guidance in assessing its severity. An example is the *Abbey Pain Scale*, which scores six observations on a scale of 1–3: vocalization, facial expression, change in body language, behaviour change, physiological state and physical changes (reference p. 239).

Pain will be best monitored by staff that work closely with the patient (as in washing, feeding or turning) and they should be encouraged to report any suspicion of pain so that it can be appropriately treated, with oral opioids if judged necessary. Whether the behaviours regarded as indicating pain have ceased or been modified can then be assessed. Some studies suggest that facial grimacing and vocalizations are accurate means for assessing the presence of pain in dementia, but not its intensity. An opioid suspension will be easier to swallow than tablets, but if swallowing is difficult, an intermittent or continuous infusion of (say) morphine with an anti-emetic is indicated.

The recognition of distress may come not only through noting a new sign or behaviour at the time of distress but also the absence of a sign or behaviour when the individual is comfortable. The observations by several carers may pick up additional signs and behaviours, and all team members should feel able to contribute to assessment.

New symptoms may indicate some reversible pathology, and a decision may be needed about whether to undertake investigations to establish a diagnosis. This may be justified only if it can be envisaged that the investigation will provide information able to guide new treatment. The question, 'What is the aim of management here?' may help limit unnecessary tests, those in which any result is not likely to bring about any change in management.

Psychological difficulties: agitation and disruptive behaviour

Agitation or disruptive behaviour should trigger a search for any underlying cause: pain, infection, a full bladder, pressure area, unrelieved constipation, a drug side-effect, perception of restraint or undue noise.

If a change in behaviour is regarded as a serious matter; tranquillizer medication should be considered, but it may increase the incidence of falls, and worsen confusion. Low-dose risperidone (1 mg/day) has improved psychotic and aggressive behaviour. Olanzapine is also commonly preferred to haloperidol because of fewer extrapyramidal side-effects:

- *risperidone 1, 2, 3, 4 mg tab.; 1 mg/ml inj.* 0.25–1 mg bd;
- *olanzapine 2.5, 5, 7.5, 10 mg tab.; 5, 10 mg wafer.* 5–20 mg/day.

Ethical issues

Usually, there will be a family member who has power of attorney to decide legal issues on behalf of the patient, and this authority may include medical decision-making. Full exchange with that person and other family members should be undertaken, and their responses to difficult options requiring decision will usually be informed by compassion and a desire to limit suffering. Issues that may arise include the following.

Is there a 'Not For Resuscitation' (NFR) order in the event of a sudden deterioration?
It is now generally accepted that resuscitation, for example, with cardiopulmonary resuscitation (CPR), is unlikely to succeed if sudden deterioration occurs in dementia, and that it is an unwise intervention causing discomfort to the patient and distress to the family. The 'NFR' order should be written by the clinician only after consultation with family members and staff, and may be better written as an order to concentrate now on 'good palliative care' as a positive instruction.

If the patient refuses food, should some artificial method of nutrition be introduced?
There is no evidence that long-term feeding provides any benefit to persons with advanced dementia. A demented patient who refuses food is dying, and should not be force fed. Tube feeding may actually increase the risk of aspiration pneumonia.

What would have been the wishes of the patient in regard to active treatment of infection (say, of bladder or lung)?
Treatment of infection with antibiotics has not been shown to prolong survival or improve comfort in advanced dementia. The use of antibiotics not infrequently causes diarrhoea or gastrointestinal upset. Only if the patient, when competent, has left a clear directive, should such therapy be considered.

Any treatment should be guided by its capacity to improve comfort.

Should transfer from an aged care institution to an acute hospital setting be arranged if a new acute illness such as pneumonia supervenes?
If it has been agreed that the primary aim for the patient in the final stages of dementia is comfort care, transfer to an acute medical setting will be quite inappropriate. Acute hospital referral too often results in inappropriate interventions: multiple investigations, intravenous (I-V) lines, naso-gastric tubes, catheters, etc. Pulmonary infection is probably more safely managed in the aged care placement, which is the patient's familiar setting, with comfort ensured by simple medical therapies and good nursing.

The maintenance of dignity

In patients with intact cognitive ability, dignity is usually well maintained, and the individual is able to withstand major physical and emotional challenges, such as feeling a burden to others, requiring assistance with bathing and toileting, lacking opportunity for privacy. But for persons with dementia there is no opportunity to face the same challenges with humour or graceful acceptance, and observers frequently judge that dignity has been lost.

Dignity for dementia patients can be maintained by simple agreed behaviours: addressing residents by the name they prefer, maintaining good hygiene, offering choices to the extent that these can be appreciated, maintaining privacy and ensuring regular and appropriate sensory-stimulating activity (on a one-to-one basis where possible), while controlling extraneous stimuli such as unnecessary noise.

THE TERMINAL PHASE

Palliation issues

Prognosis: management of incidental disease

In Alzheimer's disease, death is commonly due to stroke, cancer or renal failure, none of which will, in most instances, justify specific therapy. Swallowing is frequently impaired, increasing the risk of choking or aspiration pneumonia. Lewy body dementia has a more rapidly progressive course to death.

Specialized units for dementia care have a major focus on improving social functioning, but this becomes inappropriate in the disorder's final stages, when the patient may be mute and bed bound. There will be heavy physical nursing demands, extra time required for counselling relatives and new symptoms to address: dyspnoea, pain, fever, oral thrush and constipation being relatively common.

These symptoms will respond to routine palliative care interventions with oxygen, analgesics, paracetamol, mouth care and aperients, but it may be questioned whether treatment at this stage for pneumonia, for example, should include antibiotic therapy.

Feeding issues

In the past, it has been common to seek to maintain nutrition for a person with advanced dementia through inserting a naso-gastric tube, and to use that route for continuing the administration of medications. It is now increasingly recognized that a demented person who refuses food is dying, and it is unkind to force food upon such individuals, or to subject them to the discomfort of a naso-gastric tube. Subcutaneous (S/C) administration of medications may be necessary; feeding by per-endoscopic gastrostomy (PEG), though usually a route that is more comfortable for the patient than a naso-gastric tube, remains difficult to justify for people with advanced dementia.

Symptom recognition and management

Attending physicians are sometimes reluctant to prescribe major analgesics such as opioids, fearing questioning by family members or government authorities. Inadequate palliation of symptoms is not unusual in dementia, and a second opinion, including support from palliative care team members may be helpful. This can facilitate a culture of effective palliation that has the potential to increase staff confidence, improve morale and change practice in dementia care. If psychotic and aggressive behaviour persists at this stage of relative immobility, a continuous S/C infusion of haloperidol should be considered:

- *haloperidol 5 mg inj.* 5–15 mg/24 h.

If there is any suspicion of pain, a small dose of morphine can be added:

- *morphine 5, 10, 15 mg inj.* 5–15 mg/24 h.

Decision-making: advance directives and appointment of a proxy

Few elderly persons write advance directives, and it is important that family physicians encourage family discussion early in the course of dementia, so that, later in the illness, family members can give an honest reflection on the dying person's wishes, as far as they understand them. Most families favour the least aggressive care during the terminal phase of dementia, wishing to protect their relative from further discomfort.

If family members have been involved in discussion about management from earlier stages of the patient's decline, and been able to agree about the patient's probable wishes regarding care, they are less likely to ask for aggressive treatment.

If it can be agreed with family that extraordinary measures will not be undertaken, some discussion will be necessary concerning which interventions are accepted as extraordinary. They may include: CPR, I-V hydration, I-V antibiotics, assisted respiration and artificial feeding with a naso-gastric tube or gastrostomy.

It is best if decisions about such measures are made in advance, before the interventions are undertaken, as, once begun, it is more difficult to withdraw them without raising issues of assisting death, particularly if death is likely to occur within a short time of the withdrawal. The recording of such decisions in ways that have the support of family members, and in places where they can be accessed readily – with a close family member, with the local family physician, at the specialist neurology clinic or in the hospital case notes – is a necessary component of writing a directive well in advance of the time it may be needed.

Post-mortem examination

As indicated in the section on Creutzfeldt–Jakob disease (CJD), any case in which there has been a rapid evolution of dementia ought to be referred for post-mortem examination, since a prion infection may be impossible to diagnose during life.

5

Amyotrophic lateral sclerosis (motor neurone disease)

The two common names for this condition – amyotrophic lateral sclerosis (ALS) in the USA, motor neurone disease (MND) in the UK – are an established difficulty. For this discussion ALS will be preferred. The management of the symptoms of ALS, and particularly of the terminal stages, has received relatively little attention in many neurology texts. It was, however, the first major non-cancer diagnosis to receive the attention of palliative care units. An early text published by palliative care pioneer Dame Cicely Saunders devoted a major chapter to the care of ALS. Saunders recognized that the relatively predictable and inexorable course of ALS, and the steadily declining function of the patients made a palliative approach to symptom management highly appropriate. It also needed the same emotional support of patient and carers, and the same concern for the spiritual dimensions of suffering that she had recognized among cancer patients.

THE PALLIATIVE APPROACH

The availability of the glutamate antagonist *riluzole* promises no more than a small delay in the progress of ALS, but it will usually be gladly accepted and may seem useful for several months:

- *riluzole 50 mg tab.* 50 mg bd taken away from meal times.

Beyond that medication there is no reliable way to modify the disease, and there is a temptation for clinicians to adopt a therapeutic nihilism. The palliative care approach will focus with positive intent on the many interventions that can mitigate the major common physical symptoms of the disease, and at the same time encourage and support both patient and carers.

TELLING THE BAD NEWS OF ALS

Care towards the end of life is strongly influenced by the effectiveness of care in the earlier stages of disease. As denial of the reality of the diagnosis of ALS is a common reaction, and the desperate search for some curative intervention (no matter how 'alternative') is a natural response, it may prove difficult for a clinician to introduce the concepts of palliative care. Affected patients and their family members often will not wish to discuss anything except how they can best fight the disease.

From the time of diagnosis, however, the end stages can be predicted with some certainty (if with unpredictable timing) and it is desirable that planning for the terminal phase begins as early as possible. Where patient and family agreement to receive information about ALS can be obtained, a sensitive and compassionate introduction to the realities of what is ahead is appropriate early in the course of the illness.

This is not an easy responsibility for the concerned clinician to accept. The ready availability on web sites of vast amounts of information, at various levels of authority and accuracy, make it very likely that patient or family will have picked up at the very least a whisper of the terms 'ALS' or 'MND'. Many will quickly have become well informed about many potential horrors and discomforts that lie ahead.

The correct name of the disease should be clearly stated. If the diagnosis is left as a vague statement about a deterioration of motor nerves it may readily be confused with multiple sclerosis or one of the neuropathies. It may be helpful to assure the patient that mental function will usually be maintained and that no serious unmanageable pain should be expected. (It is legitimate to refrain from mentioning a very rare form of ALS that is accompanied by dementia.) It will be important not to say too much; a lecture on ALS is not necessary. One should allow questions, allocating a generous amount of time, and suggest opportunities to return for further discussion.

A second opinion will commonly be requested, and should be arranged.

End-of-life discussion

The ALS Workgroup of the *Robert Wood Johnson Foundation* identified six 'triggers' – events or circumstances in the progress of the illness – when it might be more possible and appropriate to initiate discussion about end-of-life issues, and raise with the patient and the family the suggestion of referral to a palliative care service.

They were:

1. a direct indication by the patient or family that they wish to raise the issues of what is ahead;
2. recognition of severe psychological or spiritual distress;
3. pain requiring increasing and high doses of analgesic;
4. swallowing difficulties requiring introduction of a feeding tube;
5. dyspnoea or symptoms of hypoventilation raising the issue of ventilatory assistance;
6. loss of function of two body regions (bulbar, arms or legs).

Advance directives (also pp. 205–206)

At some stage, during the early course of the disease, opportunity should be sought to raise the question of intrusive interventions which may need decision later on.

These include:

• assisted ventilation,
• intubation,
• artificial feeding and gastrostomy,
• the risk of complete paralysis and a 'locked-in' state.

If the opportunity to write an advance directive is available, that option can be raised. If there is interest in framing an advance directive, it is important to make clear that a written record of patient wishes on such matters need not be binding for all time. It can and should be reviewed on subsequent occasions. Where such a statement exists, and is accessible, it can prove an extremely valuable aid to the testing times for decision-making.

Supervision of care

The diagnosis of ALS will commonly be the responsibility of a neurologist, who will often continue to oversee care. In the early stages of the disease, home care is most appropriate, and can be guided by a family physician. Close networking and cooperation is desirable between the various specialities (respiratory, gastroenterology, pain management, etc.). Their interventions become increasingly important as the terminal phase approaches. A question to be answered then may be 'Who is to take overall responsibility for managing that final course'. The neurologist may not have easy access to a home care team for intensive supervision. If a palliative care unit can be involved, it may be the best resource for maintaining home care, and a hospice may offer the best final site for in-patient care.

SUPPORTIVE PHASE

Palliation issues

Muscle weakness: spasm, fasciculations, spasticity

In muscles deprived of innervation there will be weakness and wasting, fasciculations and cramps. Spasticity and the risk of contractures is less because of the relatively rapid evolution of the disease. Exercise will not in itself maintain muscle function, but in conjunction with passive movements it will defend against contractures. Mobility aids become essential, moving from walking stick to frame and wheelchair, and patients need reassurance that to use these aids is not 'giving-in' to the disease or accepting 'defeat'.

Muscle fasciculations occur early, but are rarely distressing, although they may be irritating. If necessary they may be reduced by an anticonvulsant:

- *carbamazepine 100, 200 mg tab.; 200, 400 SR tab.* 200–400 mg bd;
- *clonazepam 0.5, 2 mg tab.; 1 mg inj.* 1 mg bd;
- *quinine 300 mg tab.* 150–300 mg daily or bd.

Spasm of muscles can be severe, and may require treatment with:

- *baclofen 5 mg tab.* 10–30 mg tds.

Progressive hypoxia: assisted ventilation

Loss of power in muscles of respiration leads to sleeplessness, orthopnoea, daytime fatigue, morning headache, weight loss, syncope and dizziness, an increased risk of respiratory infection and diffuse pain in the head and neck and arms.

Non-invasive ventilation should be discussed as soon as these symptoms are recognized, and well before they become severe. A simple indication for beginning intermittent bilevel positive air pressure (BiPAP) ventilation is the onset of orthopnoea, which may be supplemented by a $pO_2 <$ 65 mmHg. A sleep study (if available) may assess best the degree of nocturnal hypoxia, and help determine when ventilatory assistance is appropriate. Provided via a close-fitting face mask, a BiPAP is usually well accepted, now being available in convenient portable models.

As deterioration continues towards the terminal phase, BiPAP will be required more consistently, up to 24 h a day. Then the question of more intrusive ventilatory support will need to be addressed.

The levels of decision-making regarding intubation for ventilatory support have been outlined earlier in the chapter on respiratory issues (p. 73).

Progressive levels of respiratory intervention will need to be considered as the weakness of respiratory muscles increases, but their implications will, ideally, have already been addressed before there is any urgent situation of deterioration to confront.

A chest infection may cause an accumulation of secretions and require insertion of a nasal or oral endotracheal tube to allow suction for their effective removal.

Such a tube cannot be left in place for very many days, nor is it suitable for repeated insertion. Therefore to allow longer-term aspiration of the bronchial passages a tracheostomy may have to be considered. Family members, once they have been given basic training, should be able to manage the regular clearing of secretions via this route in the home.

There is the additional advantage that, in persistent hypoxia, a tracheostomy may be helpful on its own for reducing some of the 'dead space' of the upper air passages.

Finally, however, it may become apparent that hypoxia can be relieved on a more permanent basis only by employing positive pressure ventilation via a tracheostomy.

Each degree of intervention is an opportunity to review again what is likely to lie ahead, and to encourage patient and family participation in anticipatory decision-making. In the absence of such thoughtful preparation, there is a risk that an acute deterioration will require urgent transfer to hospital where the performance of an emergency tracheostomy and the institution of positive pressure ventilatory support by staff who are not familiar with the patient's clinical course is an expected procedure.

There is no doubt that for many individuals with ALS, invasive ventilation via a tracheostomy can maintain life for a number of years. But care for such support is complex, and if undertaken at home causes significant strain and stress on carers. It is a common final pathway for ALS management in some countries, but in both Australia and UK it is performed far less often, and if instituted, can be withdrawn at the patient's request.

Once performed, however, it becomes very much more difficult for everyone involved to consider withdrawal of that support. It will commonly happen that, with assisted ventilation in place, the disease progresses to a stage where communication becomes quite impossible (as in locked-in syndrome). At that stage, there may be no ability to discuss adequately with the patient whether there is a wish to maintain or withdraw assisted ventilation.

In some jurisdictions (for example, in Japan), the law does not allow reversal or withdrawal of such procedures once they have been instituted, even at the expressed instruction of the patient, because that is interpreted as causing deliberate death.

This inevitably influences a clinician's decision about whether to recommend a tracheostomy in the first instance, because it is the first step towards assisted ventilation. When the law requires that, once in place, ventilation cannot be withdrawn, the family or institution are committed to a burden of care that may extend over many years.

Thick mucous airways secretions compound respiratory difficulty. Intermittent nebulized saline or acetylcysteine helps clear the bronchial passages, and manually assisted coughing techniques and vibration massage can be taught to family members:

- *acetylcysteine 20% solution.* Dilute 1:1 saline, 2–5 ml tds–qid by inhalation.

Fruits such as fresh pineapple or papaya that help liquefy the mucous should be tried. Suction of the upper airways is often uncomfortable and not very effective except via a tracheostomy. Some patients learn to use a sucker themselves to clear mouth and pharynx. Safe sucker techniques can be taught to home carers for tracheostomy care.

Speech difficulty, communication issues

Communication aids become essential as speech becomes progressively more difficult. A sense of panic can be quickly engendered when the patient is uncomfortable but is not able to make himself or herself understood. Sometimes writing will remain possible after speech can no longer be understood, using pen and paper or whiteboard; or simple reference boards with words or pictures that indicate matters needing attention.

More complex computer-based machines or light pointers moved by the head or controlled by the eyelids or eye movements are increasingly available, and spell out messages effectively (though the synthetic voices can be irritating, especially if clearly representative of the wrong gender). A speech therapist will usually help choose a suitable device, but any method will be slow, and demand considerable patience from both patient and carers.

Family members may need some guidance in their chair-side or bedside support of the patient, learning to converse with sentences that need no more than a simple response, 'yes' or 'no' able to be indicated by a blink of the eyes, perhaps.

Swallowing dysfunction

Swallowing dysfunction will benefit from the assistance of a speech therapist providing advice regarding the suitable consistency of foods to swallow, and teaching techniques to minimize the risk of aspiration. (Slow, focused feeding, lip-seal and tongue exercises to help move food in the mouth, separate swallows of tiny portions.) If swallowing difficulty progresses to a point where weight loss is very obvious, consideration must be given to the insertion of a naso-gastric tube (very uncomfortable) or a per-endoscopic gastrostomy (PEG) feeding tube (see PEG, p. 87). In progressive disease such as ALS, if a PEG is recommended, it should be introduced before respiratory function is too much compromised (lung vital capacity less than 1l) so that patient and family can discuss the option and support the decision made by the patient.

Drooling, management of secretions

Drooling of saliva that cannot be swallowed or adequately controlled by tongue and facial muscles is reduced by injected medications:

- *glycopyrrolate injections 0.2 mg inj.* 0.2–0.4 mg qid up to 2 mg;
- *atropine 600 μg inj.* 600 μg up to qid;
- *imipramine 10, 25 mg tab.* 10–50 mg at night also reduces saliva production but may make it thicker, more tenacious and more difficult to expel.

If botulinum toxin injections are available, 50 U injected into two places in each gland (both parotid and submandibular) can suppress saliva for up to 6 months.

Bladder and bowel difficulties

Bladder spasm and spasticity causing urgency and frequency may occur in the advanced stages and responds to:

- *oxybutynin 5 mg tab.* 2.5–5 mg bd or tds.

Constipation

Constipation follows from immobility and inability of weakened muscles to 'push', and in the early stages is helped by increasing the fibre content of the diet with care to maintain water content also; later, regular aperients will be needed by mouth (while the oral route is possible), or by PEG or as rectal suppositories, micro-enemata or regular enemata. Docusate and senna tablets, MgO_2 solution and solutions containing lactulose or sorbitol are commonly employed (see Constipation in Chapter 5 of Section II, p. 82).

Sleep disturbance

Sleep is commonly disturbed, partly by difficulty in altering position, partly related to psychological difficulties, and in advanced stages also by hypoxia when lying recumbent. Patients will often prefer a reclining chair for sleep; a bed which offers powered assistance in sitting up will assist, as will careful use of appropriate sedation with benzodiazepines (pp. 116–118):

• *zolpidem 10 mg tab.* 10 mg at night is less likely to inhibit respiration.

The situation may benefit from exploration of anxieties, with honest responses to questions.

Psychological difficulties: inappropriate moods

In the early phases of ALS, considerable support may be available through associations established for families and patients facing the threat of this disease; persons with common issues to discuss, and practical suggestions for care.

In one study, one third of patients with advanced ALS had considered suicide, particularly those who felt a burden to others, and were sleepless or with persistent pain and other discomforts.

The common method for entering upon psychological support is to encourage a client to talk of his or her discomfort with counsellors who are trained to *listen*. In the later stages of ALS the patient commonly must struggle to communicate the most basic needs using shorthand means that cannot express depths of feeling except, perhaps, through eyes and tears. It will be common for a patient to feel a burden to family and other caregivers; to experience enormous frustration in not being able to respond to close family and friends. This can be particularly difficult if there are children of the patient, unsure of how to approach their parent.

It may be possible to establish some simple rituals that bring considerable comfort to both carer and patient. Occasionally, these rituals may have a spiritual or religious significance – listening to a hymn together, reading from a favourite book, looking through past photographs or recalling past stories.

Often there will be just one important carer (family or friend) whose presence is most comforting, whose interpretation of patient needs is more intuitive or more experienced. That person may be able to bring to the bedside many different materials that offer meaning and support (books, music, touch, pictures, familiar stories or recollections of things shared in the recent or distant past). The provision of support for key caregivers is also an important consideration in the programme of management. To be able to call upon such individuals in difficult times can be a great assistance to professional staff.

Spontaneous inappropriate laughing or crying (sometimes termed 'false laughter') may occur (perhaps indicative of pseudo-bulbar disease) and is both an embarrassment to the patient and an interference to communication. It may be assisted by teaching the patient to deliberately change the pattern of breathing when an episode occurs. If it is judged to require treatment, consider a tri-cyclic antidepressant such as amitriptyline, or:

- *citalopram 20 mg tab.* 20–40 mg at night;
- *carbidopa 50 mg; levodopa 200 mg.* 1–2 tab. daily;
- *lithium carbonate 250 mg tab.*; 450 mg SR tab. 400 mg daily.

Pain

Pain will usually be due to inability to change posture, with painful pressure on skin points and limbs tired from sitting in one position for a long time. Muscle spasms and cramps may occur, and are best treated with baclofen or quinine (see Muscle cramps in Chapter 2 of Section II), taking care that this does not exaggerate weakness. Some patients find fasciculations irritating. Difficulty in moving muscles makes them stiff, and can lead to frozen joints (especially shoulder). Massage and gentle heat may assist, with passive movement and small doses of diazepam. Electrically operated beds help patients move position with less effort.

Dysaesthesia may be experienced, and respond best to drugs such as amitriptyline.

Skin discomfort from pressure on a single area requires regular assistance with movement, and is a common cause of pain; also parts of the body become tired and stiff through being left in one position for long periods. Transcutaneous electrical nerve simulation (TENS) machines bring relief for some patients, but require persistence and skill and for most patients prove difficult to use effectively.

Analgesics will often be necessary and may need to include Level 3 drugs of the World Health Organization (WHO) ladder (p. 99). A continuous infusion of injectable opioid (morphine, hydromorphone or fentanyl) in quite small dose, will usually bring acceptable relief.

THE TERMINAL PHASE

Palliation issues

Hypoxia and drowsiness from respiratory muscle weakness

Death in ALS occurs most often from respiratory failure. The accumulation of carbon dioxide leads to drowsiness and sleep, and the final pathway is commonly quiet and apparently free from distress. Attendants may need to make sure that the process is assisted by regular or continuous morphine infusions; anticholinergics (e.g. hyoscine hydrobromide) to reduce secretions and a benzodiazepine (e.g. midazolam) to control residual anxiety added in the one syringe.

There is accompanying hypoxia, but the use of oxygen via nasal cannulae may not improve function, or delay dying.

Pain from immobile limbs, pressure areas

The continuous subcutaneous (S/C) infusion is an everyday component of final palliation for pain control in cancer care. It also has a major place here, delivering a mix of helpful medications over 24 h, with doses titrated depending on observed responses:

- *morphine 10–30 mg* for painful limbs and tender pressure spots;
- *midazolam 5–15 mg* to lessen the pressure of a constant anxiety;
- *glycopyrrolate 0.4–0.6 mg or hyoscine 0.8–1.2 mg* to help dry pharyngeal secretions.

Accumulation of secretions

Secretions continue to accumulate in the pharynx, and while their volume maybe reduced by anticholinergic medications (see above) they may become more tenacious. Gently clearing the mouth with a swab or tissue on the finger can assist and is usually more comfortable than the use of suction.

Anxiety and fear of choking

Anxiety related to fear of pain and of choking to death has led to campaigns to make available in homes a means for delivering sedation quickly, for example a pre-loaded syringe, kept in the home refrigerator for S/C injection via an indwelling butterfly needle:

- *morphine 5–10 mg inj. + midazolam 2.5–5 mg inj.*

Such fear is understandable, but largely unfounded, because choking is rarely a cause of death, and quite direct reassurance is appropriate. Staff, as well as family members, may need assistance in accepting the responsibility to give such medication when it may possibly be the last intervention prior to death. '*You will not have caused death in giving that injection; but you will ensure that death is as free from discomfort as possible*'.

Depression and frustration

Depression and frustration are an understandable outcome of the loss of control that ALS patients experience. Irritability, anger, tearfulness or emotional withdrawal may be manifestations of this distress. These are probably best handled by trying to ensure that the greatest degree of decision-making stays with the patient, and that a patient and attentive presence is able to respond to every need that can be elicited or understood. There are no injectable anti-depressants, but a liquid presentation of a tricyclic antidepressant:

- *amitriptyline 25, 75 mg/5 ml susp.* 25–75 mg at night; or
- *fluoxetine 20 mg/5 ml susp.* 20–60 mg/day may be available, and prove useful if able to be administered through a gastrostomy. Alternatively, crushed tablets can be administered via that route.

Requests for euthanasia

Requests for euthanasia by patients with ALS are not uncommon and it may be appropriate to anticipate some direct or indirect approach of this kind; the apparently hopeless outlook and the level of disability and discomfort can make an early demise seem a desirable opportunity. Honest responses are needed, and except in the few countries where assisted suicide is permitted, will indicate what cannot be done, but also what can be done to achieve the greatest degree of comfort, with a promise to do nothing to artificially delay the approach of death (see chapter Euthanasia in Section IV, pp. 219–222).

Exhaustion and burn-out among carers

Even though the total burden of care for ALS has been described as less than for dementia (because of the usual lack of problem behaviour in ALS), the emotional drain on carers, particularly close family members, is consider-able, and they also may experience, and be willing to express, a wish that death might come more quickly to the patient, sometimes associated with a feeling of guilt or anger. It will be important to encourage discussion, to listen to feelings and clarify the several difficulties and what might be done to address them more effectively; what additional resources or respite opportunities can be called upon.

6

Incurable infections of the nervous system

The prime examples of incurable infections of the nervous system that lead to major morbidity and death are rabies, Creutzfeldt–Jakob disease (CJD) and human immunodeficiency virus (HIV). Other chronic and persistent viral infections of the central nervous system (CNS) that commonly lead to progressive deterioration and death include progressive multifocal leukoencephalopathy (PML) and subacute sclerosing panencephalitis. In these conditions, progressive cognitive impairment, seizures, myoclonus, ataxia and visual loss commonly proceed to a persistent vegetative state.

RABIES

Rabies is a uniformly fatal disease once clinical symptoms are manifest. The few who survive have received either pre-exposure prophylaxis or expeditious post-exposure prophylaxis after the rabid contact and before developing frank clinical disease. Therefore, there is a need to suspect the possibility of rabies early, and vaccinate promptly.

Rabies presents as either encephalitis or paralysis. Encephalitic or 'furious' rabies (most cases) has symptoms of hydrophobia, pharyngeal spasms and hyperactivity leading to paralysis, coma and death. The paralytic form, 'dumb rabies', is much less common.

Rabies progresses through five clinical stages with much variability, depending on extent of bites, amount of secretion encountered and proximity to the CNS; that is, disease transmitted through bites close to the brain will progress faster than disease transmitted through bites on the lower extremities.

The incubation period following the bite of an infected creature (dog, bat, etc.) ranges from 10 days to 1 year, with an average of 1–2 months.

A prodromal period occurs first, with non-specific flu-like symptoms, including malaise, anorexia, irritability, low-grade fever, headache, nausea, vomiting; paraesthesia, pain or numbness may be present at the bite site.

This is followed about a week later by an acute neurological syndrome with dysarthria, dysphagia, excessive salivation, diplopia, vertigo, nystagmus, restlessness, agitation, visual or auditory hallucinations, manic behaviour alternating with lethargy, hydrophobia associated with painful contractions of pharyngeal muscles. Deep tendon reflexes are hyperactive; positive Babinski signs and nuchal rigidity may be demonstrated.

Death will be expected about 2 weeks after onset of these symptoms, and include a stage of generalized flaccid paralysis, seizures and coma. There will be hydrophobia, prolonged apnoea, and finally respiratory and vascular collapse.

Palliation issues

Adequate sedation

In the face of a horrifying progressive fatal disease, the aim is to provide comfort for the patient and reassurance for the family, ensuring that doses of medication are adequate to prevent agitation and hallucinations in this distressing and apparently hopeless situation, and to ease the patient through to a quiet and apparently comfortable death.

Medications to provide palliation include the following, but there is no upper dose limit, dosages should be increased as necessary to achieve adequate control of discomfort:

- *propofol* 1–3 mg/kg/hourly intravenous (I-V);
- *diazepam* 10 mg inj. 5–50 mg I-V/24 h;
- *clonazepam* 1 mg inj. 2–6 mg I-V or subcutaneous (S/C)/24 h;
- *ketamine* 1–10 mg/ml inj. 100–500 mg by continuous S/C or I-V infusion/24 h.

Reduction in oral secretions

Hyoscine hydrobromide 0.4 mg inj. 1.2–2.0 mg by continuous S/C infusion/24 h will reduce oral secretions.

Continuous supervision to ensure titration of medication achieves comfort

Death usually follows 2–3 days after onset of paralysis unless it is delayed by life support with intubation and continuous sedation, or even general anaesthesia. These interventions seem unnecessary, merely deferring an inevitable finality.

CREUTZFELDT–JAKOB DISEASE

CJD is one of a number of spongiform encephalopathies in which a prion infection leads to amyloid deposits in nerve tissue, with spongy degeneration and damage to neurones, particularly in the basal ganglia, caudate nucleus and cerebellum. It has followed transplantation of dura mater or brain cells in neurosurgical procedures, but transmission from person to person is not fully understood. No transmission to attending persons has been described, but the prions can be present outside of the nervous system, and it is clearly sensible for staff and family who become closely associated with a known patient to maintain a high standard of protection against contamination by body fluids, and cerebrospinal fluid (CSF) in particular.

The diagnosis of CJD presents difficulties, being only certain when confirmed at post-mortem. It may be suspected in a case of rapidly progressive dementia with any of these clinical features: myoclonus, pyramidal signs, extrapyramidal signs, cerebellar signs or a characteristic electroencephalogram. Some cases are first recognized by the occurrence of psychiatric symptoms. Early stages of CJD also involve both generalized symptoms: confusion, memory loss, anxiety and depression; also more focal neurological signs: ataxia, visual loss, aphasia, pareses, myoclonus.

Deterioration occurs over months, survival extends occasionally to years. The combination of psychiatric disorder, loss of cognitive ability and physical disability (weakness, ataxia, choreiform movements) makes home care by families a significant burden, and indicates the need for respite opportunities and the desirability of holistic care for the final stages of the illness, most readily available in a setting supported by a recognized palliative care service.

The terminal course of CJD is well described in a father's diary, recounting early evidence of disease and inexorable and progressive deterioration in a 16-year-old youth who had received a cadaveric dura mater graft to repair a defect following removal of a cerebral tumour at the age of 2 years. The difficulty in establishing a diagnosis, and the distressing symptoms of muscle jerks and deterioration in cognition with episodes of aggression and high fever are described very movingly in simple lay terms.
(See 'A father's diary': www.fortunecity.com/healthclub/cpr/798/cjd.htm)

Palliation issues
Delirium, cognition disturbance, changes in personality, psychosis
The progress of CJD is marked initially by changes in personality and the onset of hallucinations and delusional thinking. There is an increasingly

high level of physical dependency, with major psychiatric manifestations, dementia and involuntary movements.

Myoclonus

For reducing myoclonus:

- *clonazepam 0.5, 2 mg tab.; 1 mg inj.* 0.5–1 mg bd or tds is effective.

The disease comes to its final stages quite rapidly in many instances, the patient being commonly mute, quiet and unresponsive.

A continuous S/C infusion combining:

- *clonazepam 2 mg, haloperidol 5–10 mg and morphine 15–30 mg* in a single syringe over 24 h may ensure comfort.

Neuropathic pain and dysaesthesia

Central and neuropathic pain and dysaesthesia require regular review and administration of antipsychotic and analgesic medication:

- *haloperidol 1.5–5 mg bd, carbamazepine 200–400 mg mane* and *morphine sulphate 5–10 mg 3–4 hourly prn* is appropriate.

Nutrition and hydration

Aspiration pneumonia is a risk, and issues of nutrition and hydration maybe raised, but procedures such as feeding gastrostomy or tracheostomy are not recommended. The predictable final outcome should encourage discussion of the major aim and focus of management as avoidance of discomfort rather than any measures that extend life.

Effect on carers of the inevitable nature of the disease

Family members and carers may need close support as they confront the distressing manifestations of the disease and the certain prospect of death. Anger must be expected if the infection was introduced by surgery.

Post-mortem examination. As the diagnosis of CJD in life is often unclear, a post-mortem examination will be sought in any case of rapidly progressive dementia. This ought to be anticipated and discussed in advance of death so that family members are prepared for what some will find distressing. Strict precautions against contamination must be maintained by those who perform the examination; it is therefore commonly performed only at special centres.

HIV-ACQUIRED IMMUNODEFICIENCY SYNDROME (AIDS)

The availability in developed countries of highly active antiretroviral therapy (HAART) changed the trajectory of HIV disease, extending the length of the supportive phase of care of acquired immunodeficiency syndrome (AIDS) to years and decades.

At the same time, the social setting of infected individuals changed from the gay male communities that were first to be affected in many countries. HIV infection now affects children, adolescents and adults of both sexes from many walks of life. Prison populations, the poor and injecting drug users have been described as particularly at risk.

The initial phase of HIV infection

Soon after an initial exposure to infection, many patients experience an acute viral-type illness with fever, sore throat, rash, lymphadenopathy; but some have no recognizable illness. A latent clinical period follows, with few symptoms, but viral replication is occurring and after a variable period there will be intermittent fever, weight loss, diarrhoea, rashes, lethargy and malaise. One or more complications or consequences of HIV infection, the 'AIDS-defining illnesses', remain a common way in which the disease is recognized (Table III.6.1).

The effectiveness of current therapies encourages a positive approach to treatment, characterized by therapeutic optimism. Mention of end-of-life issues, including involvement of palliative care services, may be seen as defeatist.

Nevertheless, HIV infection continues to cause death, and rates of infection are increasing rather than declining. Some individuals do not tolerate HAART well; in others substance abuse disturbs compliance and introduces additional complications (e.g. hepatitis B and C, end-stage renal disease); some are unable to accept the discipline of regular therapy. Discrimination and stigmatization of infected persons remains a problem in many settings (e.g. schools). HAART regimens are not successful for all patients; many patients find themselves facing death from AIDS at the same time that many others are having favourable responses to antiretroviral therapy. Patients and physicians have described death from AIDS in the new protease inhibitor era as having transformed from fate to tragedy.

The longer prognosis that persons receiving HAART can expect does not remove from them the anxieties related to site and process of inevitable end-of-life care or the fear of complicating illnesses that may herald the

Table 111.6.1 AIDS-defining illnesses

Opportunistic infections	Malignancies
• Oesophageal candidiasis	• Invasive carcinoma of the cervix
• Coccidiomycosis	• Kaposi's sarcoma
• Cryptococcosis	• Burkitt's lymphoma
• Cryptosporidiosis	• Immunoblastic lymphoma
• CMV	• Primary brain lymphoma
• Herpes simplex	
• Histoplasmosis	**Other conditions**
• Isosporiasis	• Encephalopathy
• Mycobacteria	• Wasting syndrome
• PCP	
• Recurrent bacterial pneumonia	
• PML	
• Salmonella septicaemia	
• Toxoplasmosis	

CMV: cytomegalovirus; PCP: pneumocystis carinii pneumonia;
PML: progressive multifocal leukoenccphalopathy.

onset of a terminal phase of the illness. Both the medical regimens required and the psychiatric issues that are associated are complex, and decisions about changes in treatment and management call for good communication and sympathetic engagement by health professionals.

Increasingly, therefore, the need is being recognized to link a palliative approach with disease-specific treatment. That approach will be particularly concerned with symptom control, points for decision-making regarding care, quality of life and issues related to carers and family members.

THE SUPPORTIVE PHASE OF HIV INFECTION

Palliation issues
Surveillance for adherence to treatment and co-morbidities
The multiple problems of established AIDS require active palliation along with preventive and active treatment for the opportunistic infections that take advantage of reduced immunity. CD_4 counts represent surface receptors on T lymphocytes, critical for defence against HIV. With HAART, CD4 counts remain higher, the viral load is kept lower and patients live longer. Fever, night sweats and weight loss are reduced and AIDS-defining illnesses are avoided. A programme of supportive care will therefore aim to ensure

good adherence to HAART and early awareness and prompt management of opportunistic infection, for example:

- cotrimoxazole for pneumocystis;
- azithromycin plus rifabutin and ethambutol for mycobacterium avium;
- fluconazole for cryptococcosis;
- ganciclovir for cytomegalovirus (CMV) (not so effective).

Any of these therapies, like the HAART drugs, may cause significant side-effects.

A constructive emotional support will be a very necessary component of care when dealing with the many patients with HIV who are vulnerable and disadvantaged individuals, living in poor circumstances and at risk of substance abuse and family dysfunction. For various reasons (e.g. drug side-effects, change in location, onset of dementia) many will stop the drug treatment and present with an AIDS-related opportunistic infection. HAART drugs interact with many other drugs employed in management. Carbamazepine for neuropathic pain, for example, should not be used in combination with a protease inhibitor.

Delirium and dementia, psychiatric issues

Many possible causes of delirium and dementia include HIV itself (encephalopathy), and infections – toxoplasmosis, primary cerebral lymphoma, CMV and neurosyphilis – may be diagnosed. Psychiatric disturbances – hypomania and schizophrenia – may require symptomatic treatment; for example:

- *haloperidol 0.5, 1.5, 5 mg tab.; 5, 50 mg inj.* 1.5–10 mg/day;
- *olanzapine 2.5, 5, 7.5, 10 mg tab.* Up to 10 mg/day; or
- *risperidone 1, 2, 3, 4 mg tab.* 0.5–2 mg orally, daily in divided doses.

Cognitive impairment and frank dementia may be more commonly observed since the advent of HAART, partly because of the longer life expectancy.

Neuropathic pain

A neuropathic element is predominant in pain, and may not be relieved by HAART; indeed in some cases the drugs may exacerbate the neuropathy. A coordinated mix of 'cure' and 'care' services is necessary to provide appropriate support during the erratic course of the disease. Peripheral neuropathy (and dry mouth) are symptoms that may arise from the effects of the disease itself or as side-effects of treatment.

Symptom management

A wide range of possible symptoms continue to threaten comfort through-out the supportive phase of care. They include diarrhoea (which may be severe), weight loss, nausea and vomiting, mouth discomfort and dysphagia, mania and hallucinations, pain and depression. Such discomforts fluctuate independent of treatment. Lipodystrophy leads to a characteristic facies and the disfigurement serves as a stigma for the disease. Diabetes and cardiovas-cular disease may be side-effects of HAART, especially the protease inhibitor drugs.

Skin problems are common and often severe. They include dry skin, seborrhoeic dermatitis, scabies, molluscum contagiosum, psoriasis, sweating, pruritus and Kaposi's sarcoma. Skin metastases and fungating tumours may occur.

Diarrhoea is a very disabling problem in HIV infection and AIDS. It occurs in up to 90% of patients at some stage. Changes of therapy may contribute. Stool examinations may establish a treatable infective cause, but HIV itself can cause diarrhoea.

Symptomatic control may use:

- *loperamide, codeine or morphine* (see Diarrhoea, pp. 84–85);
- *octreotide 50, 100 μg inj.* 50–300 μg S/C, twice daily (an expensive option).

Cough and dyspnoea are commonly due to infection; for example, pneumo-cystis carinii pneumonia (PCP), tuberculosis, CMV, *Cryptococcus neoformans*, *Nocardia* species.

Fatigue

Fatigue is quite prevalent. It relates to co-morbidities, as well as the effects of the disease itself and the medications being taken to control its progress. Sometimes attention to anaemia or depression may lead to some improvement.

THE NEED FOR CONSISTENT SUPERVISION

The disease course of treated HIV infection is marked by exacerbations and remissions, making difficult the setting of clinical goals. There are multiple possible complications and discomforts attending HIV infection, and many specialities (immunology, infectious diseases, ophthalmology, oncology, haematology, neurology, etc.) have relevant contributions to make to care.

Any one of these might assume prime responsibility for clinical management of a particular case. Continuing availability of consultation with a skilled and interested infectious disease physician is especially desirable for preservation of optimal comfort and prognosis during the supportive phase of the disease. That phase may continue for many years.

As future progress is less certain, advance directives are quite difficult to frame, but they remain very relevant to clinical decisions on goals of care. General functional status (both physical and psychological) is a better guide to prognosis than laboratory disease markers although CD4 counts are also informative.

THE TERMINAL PHASE OF HIV-AIDS

The terminal stage in AIDS may not be clearly marked. Patients may be well one day, and have a severe life-threatening infection the next day, but aggressive treatment may bring about a further stable period, even for years. New medications continue to be introduced, bringing a renewed hope of greater comfort and well-being.

There is an uncertainty regarding prognosis that is difficult for patients, family and carers. Whether aggressive treatment for infections should always be undertaken is sometimes difficult to determine. Some patients tire of taking medications, and feel their quality of life is poor. Antiretroviral agents may lose effect; the patient may not wish to prolong life. The alternative, dying, is not necessarily more comfortable, however. Uncontrolled diarrhoea, for example, may cause a very prolonged and uncomfortable death. Therefore it may be prudent to continue prophylactic treatment for opportunistic infections into the terminal stage.

Palliation issues

Transition to a palliative approach

HAART has transformed HIV infection into a manageable chronic disease, and referral for terminal care in a palliative care institution (common in at least some centres during the early years of the epidemic) is uncommon. As with other neurological diseases in which a long supportive period of care is usual, there is a difficulty in facing the transition to a terminal phase of care, and in judging when the patient's condition is such that end-of-life issues need to be addressed. Some clinicians experience that difficulty more than do patients or family members. They will be reluctant to initiate discussion about end-of-life issues unless the patient is clearly very sick, or has a very low CD4 count. But to perceive a dichotomy or even competition between 'curative' and 'palliative' approaches is unhelpful. What is required here, as elsewhere, is an integrated model that provides comprehensive care to patients and also to their families.

Suitable site of care

Despite prolonged survival, death remains a common outcome for persons infected with HIV. Many are socioeconomically disadvantaged, and have a history of drug abuse, leading to an erratic clinical course as patients take up or defect from treatment programmes. Finding a suitable site for care for a dependent, cognitively impaired patient with AIDS may present difficulties; the patient may be much younger than those admitted usually to a nursing home/aged care facility, and some institutions may be reluctant to admit AIDS patients through inappropriate discriminatory policies or staff prejudice.

Staff attitudes and protection

HIV is associated with a gay lifestyle or substance abuse. Disinhibition and cognitive deterioration may occur. Staff may perceive patients as disruptive, unwilling to follow institutional routines. Patients are often very knowledgeable about their disease, and aware of available treatments and their advantages and disadvantages. Deliberate education of staff may be necessary to assist the maintenance of a compassionate attitude, and to reassure them of the minimal danger of transmission, provided that universal precautions, to protect against contamination by body fluids, are followed.

Cognitive dysfunction and dementia

Progression of AIDS dementia may be slowed, and even reversed in some patients, with appropriate antiretroviral therapy. AIDS dementia is more common than in the early days of the epidemic, however, mainly because of the much-prolonged survival.

Pain management in drug-using patient

Pain management presents problems in the patient who has been a regular user of I-V narcotics. There is likely to be tolerance to opioids, requiring higher doses for pain control. Administering opioid by controlled-release compounds or slow infusion will deny the patient the sudden euphoria of an I-V injection, and a desire for that effect may remain. Pain in AIDS is often mixed nociceptive/neuropathic, and may require a combination of opioids and membrane stabilizing agents (p. 106). Some physicians have been reluctant to offer adequate pain medication for individuals whose past life has included I-V drug use, commonly the origin of their HIV infection.

If a patient is continuing to use illegal drugs to satisfy an addiction, the formulations and doses of medications prescribed for pain may need individual assessment, but opioids should not be withheld in the presence of pain.

Fatigue
Fatigue is a common palliative issue for HIV patients (pp. 43–46).

Multiple pathologies: malignancy, end-stage liver disease, infections
In those receiving HAART, death occurs from co-morbidities of hepatitis B and C, sepsis, end-organ failure or from malignancies of various kinds, as well as from AIDS-defining illnesses. Even in the terminal stages, symptoms from infection may arise, such as painful swallowing from candidiasis, blindness from CMV or breathlessness from PCP. These will need active treatment when they contribute to physical and emotional distress.

Anxiety and depression
Patients with advanced AIDS are usually relatively young. They may have experienced multiple losses among their friends and partners. Solidarity within the gay community may have established, for some, important and extensive carer networks, but in others, anger, despair and alienation may precipitate depression and anxiety.

Family tension
Patients affected by HIV-AIDS may have been rejected by traditional family supports, and new tensions can become evident in the final course of the disease, if alienated parents or siblings seek to re-establish contact. While the primary consideration should remain the patient's well-being and wishes, the opportunity to facilitate a renewal of broken relationships may present itself. Partners of the same sex also need the same support and respect as traditional family members, particularly if also infected with HIV.

A Management Dilemma in HIV Neurology

Progressive multifocal leucoencephalopathy (PML) is a subacute demyelinating disease of the nervous system, caused by a polyoma virus designated as JC (the initials of the first patient from whom the virus was isolated). Though uncommon, it occurs occasionally as a co-morbidity in advanced HIV infection, causing a progressive neurological deficit with hemiparesis, speech defects, cognitive dysfunction and ataxia. As the onset is insidious, patients may present with established deficits. Diagnosis is usually established on clinical grounds supported by characteristic MRI changes and confirmed by finding virus in the CSF or by brain biopsy. A change in antiviral therapy may improve some cases without achieving complete resolution of the deficits, but the outcome is unpredictable, and will not be apparent for several months. Many patients will achieve little neurological improvement and remain severely impaired, but have an improved survival, able to live for 5 years or more provided treatment is maintained. The care of demented, ataxic, dysarthric persons over long periods is a great burden to family and carers. If the treatment is ceased, death is likely to occur within a few months. Thus the patient, loved one or family is faced with the prospect of two extremely difficult decisions:

1. At the time of diagnosis, whether *to accept* treatment with the slim chance of modest improvement but residual impairment, or *to refuse* treatment and accept a very limited prognosis.
2. If treatment is begun, whether *to continue* it despite the prospect of prolonged significant disability or *to withdraw* treatment (in an otherwise well patient) and expect an early death.

As with the quandary of whether assisted ventilation can legitimately be ceased in advanced amyotrophic lateral sclerosis (ALS) or muscular dystrophy (MD), there is here a question of whether life-sustaining treatment can be ceased and the patient be allowed to die. It would be unusual that an advanced directive had been prepared that was relevant to this situation, and the cognition of the patient may be so greatly impaired that (unlike ALS or MD) no informed request can be obtained from the patient. It is a situation in which the writing of a power of medical attorney document, transferring authority over such a decision to another person, could be advantageous. It would allow an assessment of the capacity and quality of life of the patient to be considered in consultation with an individual who has the best interests of the patient at heart, and foster also a clear appreciation of the personal, emotional and financial context within which the continuation or cessation of treatment should be judged.

7

Muscular dystrophy

There are many variants of muscular dystrophy, most of them quite rare. The more common types go by names such as myotonic muscular dystrophy, facioscapulohumeral muscular dystrophy, myotonic dystrophy and duchenne muscular dystrophy (DMD) and have many similar features, primarily limb, trunk and neck weakness with impairment of mobility and respiration, but sometimes also cardiac abnormalities or cataract that will need other specialist opinion. DMD is chosen as the basis for this discussion. It is first diagnosed in childhood, when increasing difficulty is observed in running, getting up from the floor and walking up stairs. By the teenage years, many will be wheelchair bound, coping with repeated chest infections, dyspnoea and night hypoxia as ventilation becomes increasingly impaired. There may be concomitant cardiac failure and intellectual disability.

THE SUPPORTIVE PHASE OF CARE

The course of DMD will commonly extend for longer than a decade, and constitutes a major burden of care for a family, usually the mother. During this time there will be continuing efforts to encourage the fullest possible life in the face of progressive muscular weakness, calling upon the advice and assistance of many health professionals for hydrotherapy, physiotherapy, speech therapy, psychotherapy and provision of special equipment.

A discipline of regular passive stretching exercises to prevent contractures, supervision of prescribed periods of standing, fitting of night plasters or consideration of tendon lengthening procedures all make demands on family members, who often become very involved, feeling a responsibility for holding back the progress of the disease. Other siblings in a family can feel that their concerns have had to be put aside. Marital conflict and divorce is sometimes an outcome of the stress experienced in the home.

For parents, after years of making sure that the patient is surrounded by positive and encouraging supports, and helping maintain best function and length of life in the face of progressive deterioration, it is difficult to accept the inevitability of the final outcome. Looking ahead to the terminal phase will be viewed by many as destructive, negative thinking.

Much of the early care and support extended to the patient and family will have been based in a paediatric setting. Increasingly, supportive care has allowed patients to survive into the third decade, and at some stage transition to supervision by an adult service will be recommended. This can be a cause of great anxiety because of separation from well-known facilities and staff on the paediatric side, increased by the adult neurologist's lack of familiarity with parent–child issues – patient dependency, surrogate decision-making and long experience in the supervision of care. If staff of the paediatric service have not been open in their acknowledgement of the grave prognosis, the adult service may feel they have been left unfairly with the responsibility to supervise the terminal course, and the patient and family may feel abandoned.

Recurrent respiratory infections are common causes of acute hospital admission, and can lead to a dependency on hospital and hospital staff. Cardiac complications occur, requiring electrocardiographical (ECG) evaluation of the risk of a conduction block and consideration of the use of a pacemaker.

Care usually will be being provided at home, and it has been suggested that to manage the death of a child or young adult with muscular dystrophy in the home can reduce the intensity of grief reactions, depression and marital difficulties commonly experienced by parents and family members.

TRANSITION TO THE TERMINAL PHASE: THE ISSUE OF VENTILATION

A key point of decision for these patients will centre on the question of assisted ventilation. This should be aired and discussed well before the time when exacerbations of infection and hypoxia are likely to precipitate an emergency admission to hospital. If that occurs, a hospital team focused solely on improvement in the immediate situation may be tempted to opt for urgent tracheostomy. A sequence of assistance introduced more gradually is preferable, starting with bilevel positive air pressure (BiPAP) assistance for nocturnal ventilation (which will prevent the headaches caused by night hypoxia), then using BiPAP to assist ventilation throughout 24 h. Finally, when BiPAP seems insufficient, tracheostomy will need to be considered. Such a sequence, leading inevitably to tracheostomy, may be considered mandatory in some countries; in others it is a matter of patient choice and clinical decision, and any step in the progress may be rejected. Even BiPAP has been described as making the suffering longer, and in Australia and UK tracheostomy for the final stage of care for DMD is relatively uncommon.

The care of a tracheostomy is a major burden for carers; it requires additional equipment for home use, and a team of individuals confident in care of the equipment and suctioning of the trachea, day and night. Suction is an uncomfortable procedure, and tracheostomy prevents speech. Many patients will prefer non-invasive supports for their convenience, comfort and maintenance of speech.

The whole question of ventilatory support is therefore a setting for the consideration of advance directives, but any foreshadowing of intentions and wishes will need the fullest discussion of options and potential risks and benefits, with information offered honestly and clearly, and without implied direction.

Palliation issues

Hypoxia, dyspnoea and headache

Hypoxia is associated with headache and a feeling of suffocation and panic. These symptoms are readily relieved by small doses of an opioid, morphine being preferred, and administered either as oral suspension, subcutaneous (S/C) bolus or continuous infusion, in whatever dose brings relief and rest from panting:

- *morphine 1, 2, 5 mg/ml susp.; 5 mg/ml inj.* 5 mg by mouth; or
- *morphine 5, 10 mg inj.* 2 mg by S/C injection is a common starting dose. With the drive to breathe quietened, an increase in carbon dioxide retention brings its own sedation.

Anxiety

The addition of a small dose of benzodiazepine will lessen anxiety and reduce the drive to fight against feelings of tiredness. Both benzodiazepines and opioids have a reputation of depressing respiratory drive, but in this situation of chronic and progressive respiratory failure it is exactly that action that will bring relief:

- *diazepam 2, 5 mg tab.* 2–5 mg bd by mouth;
- *midazolam 5, 15 mg inj.* 5–15 mg/24 h by infusion.

Such an approach can be readily accepted by many patients and families provided that they have been given sufficient support to recognize the reality of the terminal phase, and have been able to endorse the aim of best comfort rather than greater length of life at all costs.

Pain

Apart from headache, pain may be caused by pressure on the skin of immobile areas or by movement of stiffened joints. Again, small doses of opioid are an appropriate means of palliation, but carers will need reassurance that this is given for comfort and not to shorten life.

Site of care, home, hospital admission, respite

Care of a young person with muscular dystrophy at home is commonly seen as providing care in the best site. However, repeated admissions for acute management of respiratory infection is a common need, and though unsettling, may provide intermittent respite opportunity for those undertaking home care, the physical and emotional burden of which is often enormous.

Facing the terminal phase

As the condition worsens, the family may be motivated to consider a less intensive management of infection in the home, and even an acceptance that death may occur in the home. It may involve also a consideration of whether assisted ventilation might be removed, and death allowed to occur. These will usually be very difficult issues for family members to raise, though some patients themselves will have thought to raise them quite early in the course of the illness, as its progressive course becomes apparent. An advance directive on such a matter is, however, uncommon. If discussion is sought, the opportunity for palliation can be offered through the terminal phase, overcoming discomforts with a continuous infusion of sedation and analgesia (see chapter Amyotrophic Lateral Sclerosis in this Section, p. 155).

Bereavement issues

A condition which has subsumed the focus and activity of a family for many years will eventually come to its inevitable close, with a huge change in family life that may be received as a relief but also bring a void filled with grief.

The family which has managed a long course of care for a young person with muscular dystrophy is particularly vulnerable to grief. It may be slow to resolve and prone to pathological expression. Part of the programme of care for these patients ought to be a deliberate follow-up of family members to identify any abnormal grieving and recommend appropriate interventions and support.

Genetic counselling

As this genetically determined condition will often not be diagnosed until a child has grown beyond infancy, more than one child may be affected in the one family. This compounds the burden of care and of grief, and the potential second sufferer will be very aware of what lies ahead. Genetic counselling will usually be essential to support families through decisions about further pregnancies.

8

Neuropathies

Among the many causes of peripheral neuropathy are diabetes, drug side-effects, human immunodeficiency virus (HIV) infection, leprosy, vitamin deficiency, alcohol abuse and inherited nerve disorders. Very often the underlying pathology is reversible if an underlying cause can be removed, a peripheral nerve having the potential to regenerate over many months. In the interim, and sometimes indefinitely, discomforts must be treated symptomatically. Consequences such as Charcot joints and plantar ulcers may be seen if the distal limb sites are not protected from damage. Autonomic neuropathy causes syncope, bladder atony, anhidrosis and dry mouth. Persistent and severe neuropathic pain requires trial of the response to one or more of the range of drugs in the classes antidepressants, anticonvulsants and antidysrhythmics (pp. 106–107).

Guillain–Barre (GBS) is an acute onset radiculo-neuropathy that is commonly triggered by an infection, *Campylobacter jejuni* being the most frequent antecedent pathogen.

Cases of GBS commonly progress quickly, but many recover equally quickly. Treatment may be unnecessary in those who are able to walk during the second week of illness, but observation until approximately the 8th day seems appropriate to be certain that the illness does not progress. Mild cases of GBS are likely never to come to the attention of a neurologist. Severe GBS, especially in older people, is often associated with profound wasting and persisting joint immobility. Symptoms are very variable, depending on the mix of peripheral nerves mainly affected, and the severity may range from very mild, needing no treatment, to major disability with the risk of respiratory failure. Fulminant disease in GBS requires early treatment before axonal dysfunction becomes irreversible, and in many cases monitoring in an intensive care setting is recommended, ready to initiate intubation and ventilation; there is also a risk of cardiac dysrhythmia. Treatment with plasma exchange or intravenous (I-V) gamma globulin will usually ensure a favourable outlook in what is potentially a self-limited disease.

Chronic idiopathic demyelinating peripheral neuropathy (CIDP) involves similar symptoms but at a much slower rate of progression and with relapses and remissions. Treatment is usually by the administration of I-V gamma globulin. Some patients require corticosteroids as well and others need plasma exchange. Rarely, immunosuppressive agents such as azathioprine, mycophenolate and so on may be prescribed in refractory cases. Many achieve some degree of recovery with relatively minor persistent disability.

Polyneuropathies that progress slowly (over years) are most likely to be genetically determined, and usually affect motor function rather than sensory elements.

In a few cases major sequelae will require prolonged rehabilitation with mobility aids, and management of persistent pain is an occasional need.

Palliation issues
Painful neuropathy
Pain is the major discomfort of neuropathy. Nerve fibres are commonly affected according to axon length, and symptoms will typically start in peripheral areas: toes and lower legs, later tips of fingers. Initially a tingling or burning sensation accompanied by loss of sensation (often compared with walking on cotton wool or walking on stumps) it may proceed to spontaneous pain with dysaesthesia making even light touch uncomfortable. Occasionally persistent nerve pain will occur in association with a progressive sensory or sensori-motor axonal polyneuropathy. The full range of medications that assists control of neuropathic pain may be needed; no single agent will be predictably helpful. Start with tricyclic antidepressants, and add anticonvulsants or antidysrhythmics depending on response (see Neuropathic pain in Chapter 7 of Section II, p. 105).

Joint and skin damage from lack of sensation
Charcot joints and plantar ulcers may present through peripheral nerve damage and insensitive joints and feet. Palliative management includes foot care, attempts at weight reduction, careful fitting of shoes and orthotic supports.

Weakness of the extremities
Leg weakness is also an early symptom ('rubbery legs'), but it may proceed to facial and bulbar weakness with involvement of cranial nerves (see chapter Bulbar Symptoms in Section II, p. 65). Patients will need physiotherapy assistance with sticks, crutches or walking frames; simple light wrist splints

may be useful to support hand and finger movement. Occupational therapists will advise on the form of utensils and tools best suited to a particular disability.

Multiple ancillary symptoms

Reactive depression is frequent. Deep venous thrombosis is a risk. Autonomic instability commonly leads to hypotension and occasional cardiac dysrhythmia. Sexual activity is impaired, and sildenafil may assist erectile dysfunction.

Anxiety related to genetic issues

Hereditary sensory-motor neuropathy has a wide range of manifestations, with an onset in childhood being very suggestive of inherited basis. No therapies will prevent its onset or delay its progression and there may be involvement of auditory and visual function.

A family so affected may experience anxiety and guilt about having brought an affected child into the world, and it is desirable that genetic counselling for other family members and adequate supportive care for parents and child are available.

9

Huntington's disease

This neurodegenerative disease is inherited as an autosomal dominant, the genetic defect lying in the expansion of a CAG repeat on the short arm of chromosome 4. The extent of the expansion of the repeat determines the manifestations of the disease (where there are more than 40 repeats onset of the disease is certain, with fewer repeats there may be carrier status but no occurrence of the disease in that individual). Since finding the gene for Huntington's disease, it has become possible to identify those individuals who will develop the condition. That gives an especial poignancy to management, since persons so identified are often well aware of the future course of the disease with its devastating spectrum of movement disorder, psychiatric manifestations and cognitive impairment.

The symptoms of Huntington's disease usually appear first between the ages of 30 and 50 years, and progress slowly but inexorably, over a period of some 20 years or more. No known treatment prevents the disease onset or slows its progression. It is, of all diseases, one for which, from its earliest stages, palliation of symptoms is the only therapy; what needs to be considered is at what stage it can be accepted by patient and family that they are in 'palliative care'.

The variable spectrum of decline in function over time can be arbitrarily divided into five progressive stages extending over many years:

1. The time of early diagnosis when full capacity is maintained.
2. A phase in which some assistance is required but life at home is quite manageable, and continued employment may also be possible.
3. After several years, the capacity to undertake activities of daily living begins to become impaired, and regular physical assistance and emotional support is required. If that is available, home care remains quite feasible. It is at this stage that a palliative approach to care begins to be most relevant, building a team support which offers a comprehensive set of skills in assessment and management of the

many physical and psychiatric difficulties which are now becoming established and will be expected to worsen over time.

4. A further phase may become apparent only 20 years or more after the disease onset. Impairment in ability to manage daily activities is now such as to make home care much more difficult for family members (even with considerable professional support).

5. A final stage when all the resources of a total care facility are necessary.

SUPPORTIVE CARE OF HUNTINGTON'S DISEASE

Palliation issues

Various palliative issues are as follows:

1. *Issues of consent and confidentiality*: The right to know; the right not to know. There may be, for example, a grandchild who wishes to know the risk for her of developing the disease, but has a parent who does not wish to know.

2. *Financial issues*: The opportunity to access Life Insurance and Superannuation may be denied unless tests indicate an absence of the genetic markers of the disease. Loss of the ability to work raises major financial considerations.

3. *Site of care*: The most suitable site of care in advanced stages of the disease may be at home, but this makes very great demands of family members. If it is to be a nursing home, that will need to be specially equipped to offer appropriate care to individuals who are often younger than the usual aged population.

4. *Protection*: Thought must be given, in matters of safety and the environment, to the danger that sufferers are to themselves and to others (including family members, children and medical staff) through impulsive behaviour.

5. *Wish to suicide*: The wish to suicide is understandable and possibly not infrequently carried out, though affected persons know that the medical profession is prohibited from offering assistance.

6. *Feeding difficulties*: Whether to introduce a feeding tube when swallowing becomes greatly impaired is a matter calling for careful discussion with family members.

7. *Advance directives*: Raising the question of advance directives, prior to the loss of ability to write them, will at least offer an opportunity for discussion about what lies ahead.

8. *Social and family issues*: The availability of special support groups to assist with home care, counselling and decision-making. The loss of

the ability to parent a child, and the need for long-term institutional care may both cause tension and anxieties within the family and benefit from further discussion with a social worker.

Many issues from this long list need to be discussed as early as is practicable in the course of the illness, but already the patient may lack insight or have developed a psychiatric morbidity. The need to consider such matters places great demands on family members because of the genetic associations of the disease. Personality difficulties may be an early indication of the onset of the disease and cause considerable family strain. There will be a fear and a recognition that other family members may be fated to develop the condition, and the necessity to live in doubt is a significant strain. Genetic testing is available to indicate the risk of developing Huntington's disease, but some individuals will prefer not to know what might be bad news. Even when a test is negative there may be a residual 'survivor guilt'.

Exaggerated responses to anaesthetic agents (sodium pentothal and succinylcholine) have been described, causing complexity for any proposed anaesthesia for a required procedure (e.g. dental work).

The role of support organizations can be very important, allowing access to information and understanding based on the experience of other family members facing similar issues of care. Many regions will have such a focus, able to refer families to appropriate counselling and to interested medical and social supports. The internet offers a wide variety of sites where family members can learn about the condition and link with support services around the world.

THE TERMINAL PHASE

Palliation issues
Motor disorders, chorea, gait impairment

The major symptoms of Huntington's disease fall within the triad of 'dyskinesia (motor), dementia (cognition) and depression (psychological)'. They include impaired control of gait, voluntary movement and emotional reactions. In everyday social settings these manifestations may be attributed to drunkenness or psychosis, and cause embarrassment and great distress. In the advanced stages of the disease disordered movement interferes with hygiene and care. The situation of the patient evokes a horrified concern in observers, and the need to decrease the velocity and amplitude of involuntary movement is a major concern. In juvenile patients bradykinesis and dystonia may be treated with carbidopa and levodopa (see chapter Parkinson's Disease and Related Disorders in this section).

The need for transfer to an institution will usually be determined by the onset of marked limitation of mobility and gait impairment. Once admitted to a nursing home most individuals with Huntington's disease stay a long time – usually several years, and often until death. As the final phase approaches, there is progressive loss of volitional movement and impulsive involuntary movements of increasing amplitude occur:

- *tetrabenazine 25 mg tab.* 25–100 mg bd; or
- *clonazepam 0.5, 2 mg tab.; 1 mg inj.* 2–4 mg over 24 h may reduce the distress caused by these movements.

Skin sores from ceaseless movement and knocking into objects may become infected, and emphasize the need for vigilant protection.

Creating a safe environment

A safe environment has open spaces, wide doorways and no items that can be knocked over or stumbled into. Padding of protruding objects reduces skin damage through sudden uncontrolled limb movement. Beds allow for major choreiform movement and minimize the risk of falling out. To nurse a patient on a mattress on the floor is an acceptable alternative, or to have a monitor in the mattress so that it sounds a warning if a weight is no longer on it.

Depression, hallucinations, aggressive and psychotic behaviour

It is understandable that depression and thoughts of suicide plus attempts to effect it arise (in up to 30% of all cases). Psychotic episodes with hallucinations and delusions are commonly encountered. There is emotional irritability, and frequent violent outbursts, or behaviours that are difficult to tolerate without some form of constraint. Dementia in Huntington's disease is more likely to be manifest as aggressive behaviour. Regular sedation may be required to control it:

- *clonazepam 0.5 mg tab.; 1 mg inj.* 1 mg bd; or
- *lorazepam 2 mg tab.* 2–4 mg daily.

The use of antipsychotic medications will make care more manageable and reduce apparent patient distress. Atypical antipsychotic drugs are favoured over more traditional medications:

- *olanzapine 2.5, 5, 10 mg tab.; 5, 10 mg wafer.* 5–15 mg daily;
- *citalopram 20 mg tab.* 20–40 mg daily;
- *risperidone 1, 2, 3, 4 mg tab.,1 mg/ml inj.* 1–4 mg daily.

Other drugs that assist include fluoxetine, nortriptyline and haloperidol:

- *amisulpride 100, 200, 400 mg tab.* 100–200 mg bd;
- *tetrabenazine 25 mg tab.* 25–100 mg bd. are also effective in reducing the severity of chorea.

Dementia

Cognitively, affected individuals become increasingly slow in responses, with impaired learning and inability to plan. They will need to be guided through simple tasks, and eventually need full dementia care (pp. 152–154). Difficulties occur with hygiene and sleep. There is value in establishing regular routines.

Feeding difficulties

Nutrition is compromised by inability to swallow, by movements interfering with feeding and by impaired cognition. Choking is common, and leads to great anxiety in relation to meals (that may be assisted by a dose of lorazepam before eating). Frequent small meals will maintain nutrition best, with removal of distractions. There should be careful preparation of the furniture used for meals to maintain an upright posture after swallowing; thickened fluids are more readily swallowed, changing the shape of the cups used may assist, carers need to check that the mouth is empty. The insertion of a per-endoscopic gastrostomy (PEG) may be considered.

Terminal events

With poor food intake, there is weight loss. Respiratory distress occurs as muscles of respiration lose strength and coordination, and respiratory infection is a likely complication and mode of death. It will often be appropriate *not* to offer active antibiotic treatment. Fatigue and sleepiness become more marked, and the sufferer is confined to bed. At the end stage, patients are mute and rigid, finally succumbing to a combination of inanition, exhaustion and infection. Skin care at this stage will focus on the need to protect against pressure ulceration.

10

Cerebral neoplasms

Apart from a small percentage of benign tumours (most meningiomas and pituitary adenomas) neoplasms of the central nervous system are progressive and not curable. Initial management with surgery or radiotherapy (and sometimes chemotherapy) will often lead to a resolution of symptoms for a variable period, but cure cannot be promised, and a recurrence of tumour is virtually inevitable.

Cerebral metastases from tumours elsewhere are more common than primary brain malignancies. They occur in about 20% of adult cancer cases, and are more often multiple, with more widely dispersed neurological manifestations than the solitary brain lesions. However, resection of solitary metastases may be performed to combat the threat of distressing cerebral symptoms, and can provide a window of good function and hope not dissimilar to resection of a primary tumour.

Secondary spread of cancers from other parts of the body is also the most likely cause of tumours in the epidural space and spinal leptomeninges.

Effective management of symptoms should be a consistent aim throughout the course of the illness, and will become the central aspect of care as recurrences and deterioration occur. It will be important to try to prepare the family for this inevitable terminal stage as early as possible, not spelling out the worst possibilities, but recruiting their interest in reporting changes in affect or function, and helping them feel that they have permission to ask any questions about what lies ahead and about how their coping may be enhanced.

Although knowledge of the tumour histology and extent offers useful guidance, the progress of decline is often variable, including that of the terminal stage.

THE SUPPORTIVE PHASE

Palliation issues

Personality and cognitive change

Loss of clarity of thought, change in personality, physical disability, loss of independence and changes in family roles and functioning make both home care and institutional support stressful and onerous. Formerly cheerful and cooperative individuals may become morose and irritable, or exhibit obsessive fixations, paranoia or a persistent restlessness.

Some patients become unduly drowsy with slowed physical and intellectual responses; they may be helped by regular methylphenidate:

- *methylphenidate 10 mg tab.* 10–20 mg morning and midday.

Others are constantly moving, restless and anxious and will benefit from major tranquillizer assistance:

- *haloperidol 0.5, 1.5, 5 mg tab.; 5 mg inj.* 2.5–5 mg tds;
- *chlorpromazine 10, 25, 100 mg tab.; 25 mg/ml inj.* 50–200 mg tds;
- *thioridazine 10, 50, 100 mg tab.; 10 mg/ml susp.* 10–50 mg tds.

Cognitive changes cause much frustration, the patient often being aware of an inability to make sense and perform satisfactorily and the attendants finding it necessary to guess at needs and make decisions without opportunity to consult. Other possible causes of altered cognition should be checked (drugs, metabolic upsets, infection, depression).

Consequences of treatment: radiotherapy, chemotherapy, corticosteroids

Radiotherapy for cerebral tumour is often an unpleasant experience, usually being conducted over several weeks, and causing severe tiredness, not infrequently with nausea and headache. The first fractions may cause a slight exacerbation of symptoms, even though steroids are being continued. The timing of benefit cannot be predicted with confidence, sometimes being obvious within a few days, sometimes causing slow improvement only after some weeks. Late complications of radiotherapy, which can cause major damage to nerve tissue, are not seen for months to years later, and are rarely relevant in the management of cerebral tumour. If chemotherapy is employed, its common consequences of nausea, hair loss, proneness to bleeding and infection must be anticipated.

Corticosteroids are administered in doses of up to 12–16 mg of dexamethasone per day (sometimes higher doses are necessary), and inevitable side-effects will result, with altered self-image, weight gain, fragile skin prone to tears and bruising, and proximal myopathy which further reduces mobility often already compromised by paresis and incoordination. Cushingoid side-effects will appear, with changes in facial appearance, facial hair and acne. Irritability, euphoria and occasionally frank mania can occur. Occasionally, steroids trigger frank diabetes, and unusual thirst or polyuria should signal a need to test blood glucose levels. Oral hypoglycaemics or regular insulin may be required if it is felt that steroid medication should continue. Oral thrush is a common association; the mouth should be checked regularly and treated promptly.

Headache

Headache may be relieved by simple non-opioid analgesics (paracetamol) and will also be helped by corticosteroids. Morning headache with nausea is commonly regarded as indicating a cerebral tumour, but in many cases of cerebral tumour discomfort more closely resembles tension headache. If there is severe persistent headache, the use of opioid analgesics is entirely justified, following World Health Organization (WHO) ladder guidelines.

Raised intracranial pressure from cerebral oedema or obstructive hydrocephalus classically causes headache, worse in the morning, and sometimes described as increasing with coughing and bending. Vomiting on waking in the morning and (less commonly) seizures may also occur. Evidence of raised intracranial pressure indicates the need for steroid therapy, and dexamethasone is favoured, usually starting in a dose of 16 mg/day, reducing to 4 mg/day as symptoms regress.

Seizures

Seizures are reported to occur at some stage in up to 40% of cases. It is not necessary to institute prophylactic treatment in those who have never had a seizure, as anticonvulsants have significant potential side-effects (drowsiness, rashes, etc.), but both the family members and support staff should be prepared with awareness of the risk, and competent first-aid responses (lying the patient on one side and maintaining the airway). After only one seizure, anticonvulsant medication is usually begun; if there are recurrent seizures that are difficult to control, the family may be helped by instruction in appropriate measures for aborting a seizure:

- *diazepam 10 mg inj.* 10 mg delivered rectally via a syringe;
- *clonazepam 2.5 mg/ml solution.* 2.5–7.5 mg placed sublingually via a syringe.

Thromboembolism

Patients with a cerebral tumour are more prone to thromboembolism than the general population, not just because of reduced mobility, but through changes in fibrinolysis induced by tumour factors. Any signs of peripheral thrombosis should be monitored regularly, and consideration be given (taking into account an increased risk of haemorrhage) to anticoagulant therapy, perhaps best provided with daily enoxoparin injections rather then oral warfarin:

- *enoxoparin 20, 40, 60, 80, 100 mg prefilled syringe.* 1 mg/kg daily subcutaneous (S/C) injection.

Leptomeningeal spread

Tumour metastases to the leptomeninges and spinal cord cause a range of discomforts, notably pain, particularly from cranial or spinal nerve roots, and accompanied by local signs of weakness and numbness. Corticosteroids are helpful, and foci of local disease may respond well to limited radiotherapy.

THE TERMINAL PHASE

Palliation issues

Site of care

The care of a somnolent, cushingoid and weak individual, communicating with difficulty, and often irrational, is a major nursing challenge, and it may persist for weeks and months. If home care is to be maintained, a lot of equipment will be necessary to lessen the physical strain of lifting, turning and toileting a heavy patient who is unable to cooperate.

Nursing support and equipment in the home

A hospital bed with electric power, a lifting machine, an air mattress and an indwelling urinary catheter will often be necessary. Support of family by regular (at least daily) nurse visits will lift some of the burden of hygiene routines and allow discussion of progress.

Respite for carers

Periods of respite for home carers, either through providing additional home nursing (e.g. for several nights in a row) to rescue family members from sleep deprivation, or through brief admission to hospital, may allow the greater amount of terminal care to be managed in the home.

Personality change and agitation

Change in personality as well as deterioration in physical and cognitive ability causes carer distress. *'He is not the man I married'* may be heard. The establishment of a confiding relationship with a trusted professional (nurse or doctor) to allow ventilation of such feelings may relieve some of the associated sadness, guilt and anger.

Control of seizures

In the final stages, oral medications may not be swallowed predictably, and protection against seizures is best maintained by regular bolus injections or infusion of clonazepam:

- *clonazepam 0.5, 2 mg tab.; 1 mg inj.* 1–2 mg bd, or a continuous S/C infusion (2–4 mg/24 h).

Final decisions: ceasing medications (e.g. steroids), nutrition and hydration

Open and honest reflections on progress will assist in deciding such issues as:

- Cessation of unnecessary oral therapies as swallowing becomes difficult.
- Whether to continue corticosteroids.
- When to accept that patient wishes and instructions are no longer always appropriate and may need to be overridden.
- How intensively to maintain nutrition when swallowing has become difficult.
- Whether to use simple hydration with S/C infusions.

Supportive medication can be continued by bolus injection or continuous infusion if swallowing is impaired. This can be a time to assess what drugs are really useful. To cease corticosteroids may help abort a long drawn-out saga of care that offers no prospect of improvement. An attending physician can feel justified in recommending a reduction and cessation of corticosteroids when the drug is no longer, even in higher doses, maintaining lucidity, consciousness or comfort. An explanation that to withdraw the drug is not to 'kill' the patient, but may allow the natural process of the disease towards death to take its effect, will usually be accepted by family members. On the other hand, if there is evidence of persistent headache it can be appropriate to continue quite high doses of steroids through to the time of death and to provide analgesia and sedation with a continuous infusion:

- *morphine 10, 15, 30 mg inj.; midazolam 5 mg inj.* Morphine 10–50 mg + midazolam 5–15 mg over 24 h.

If agitation or restlessness continues to be a problem:

- *phenobarbitone 200 mg inj.* 200–600 mg by bolus S/C injections over 24 h; or
- *propofol 200, 500, 1 g vial.* 10 mg/h via an intravenous (I-V) line can be considered.

A patient with cerebral tumour who is no longer able to swallow will usually have a reduced level of consciousness and will not experience either hunger or thirst. If maintenance of hydration is considered, it will be primarily for the benefit of family who are finding it difficult to accommodate to the deterioration in progress. They can be gently assured of the patient's comfort, and the lack of evidence that maintaining a S/C infusion (of 1 l/24 h normal saline) affects survival at all.

11

Sequelae of traumatic brain injury

Traumatic brain injury is a major cause of disability and death in most advanced nations, and an increasing problem in virtually all developing nations, whether from motor vehicle accident or gunshot injury. In some series, approximately one third of those injured recover completely, one third are left with significant disability, and one third either die at the time of injury or soon after, or are left in a persistent vegetative state.

The management of traumatic brain injury is initially the responsibility of the intensive care physician and the neurosurgeon, and it will be uncommon for either the neurologist or the palliative care physician to be asked to consult on such cases. In particular cases where unusual sequelae supervene, a neurological opinion may be sought.

THE SUPPORTIVE PHASE

Palliation issues
Site of care
Immediate intervention commonly involves tracheostomy and intensive care supervision. The long-term support of brain-injured individuals is more commonly a responsibility for rehabilitation teams rather than neurologists. Established brain injury is for life, and the best results of rehabilitation appear to be through continued supervision by multi-disciplinary rehabilitation teams able to support an individual over a prolonged period.

Financial matters
The best site for management of the patient may be affected by financial constraints; for example whether insurance compensation for injury is applicable. Rehabilitation may be necessary over months and years, requiring

regular professional supervision or institutional care. Physical, cognitive, behavioural and psychological changes may vary, depending on the areas of the brain that are damaged.

Cognitive and psychological impairments

Persons with major head and spinal injuries are often young and have lived active, sometimes rebellious lives. Family expectations and contexts will differ markedly from those of older individuals affected by stroke, and rehabilitation requirements will differ also. Nevertheless, the physical disabilities are similar: there may be memory impairment, affective disorders, post-traumatic epilepsy, post-traumatic psychosis, depression and dementia. Individuals may lack insight, and repeatedly attempt tasks that are beyond them. There may be impulsiveness, and lack of inhibition and poor control of emotions.

Multiple symptoms: urinary, bowel, seizures, pain, disturbed sleep, skin ulcers

Complications of injury include urinary tract infections, bowel incontinence, decubitus ulcers, urolithiasis and neurological deterioration with an increased risk of seizures. Bladder and bowel dysfunction constitute a moderate to severe life problem, as does sexual dysfunction. Spastic paralysis causes marked functional impairment. Pain is predominantly neuropathic. Fatigue, constipation, ankle oedema, joint and muscle problems, and disturbed sleep are common complaints.

Caregiver fatigue

Caregivers commonly neglect their own needs, feeling a personal responsibility compounded by the judgement that no one else really understands the injured person or can give the same level of care. The long period of rehabilitation is a huge burden for family members, and the availability of support groups can be very valuable, linking with others who appreciate the risk of depression, frustration and anger in the daily round, and who can offer tips on managing common problems related to feeding, or management of urinary and bowel function.

THE TERMINAL PHASE

Palliation issues

Causes of death

An individual who has suffered a severe head injury that results in gross impairment of consciousness and a bed-fast existence, is prone to respiratory and urinary infection, and an increased risk of sepsis from pressure ulcers. Infection is a common mode of death.

Withdrawal of life support

Many, however, will have a prolonged vegetative state. After a period of 12 months, it can be gently suggested that any chance of recovery has passed, and consideration must be given to withdrawal of the nutrition and hydration that is maintaining such life as remains. Decision-making issues arise, because there usually will be no advance directive in place whereby the patient has left instruction concerning such a situation.

Guardianship issues

If family members are unsure that they have authority to authorize withdrawal of treatment there may be opportunity for them to approach a public body such as a Guardianship Board that can confirm them in that role.

Support of family members

Family members will need repeated opportunities to consider, discuss and return to the reality of the patient's plight. They should not be hurried, or given any sense that considerations like the cost of care, or the need for the bed to be available to another patient, are influencing staff advice.

Sedation during life-support withdrawal

Advice on palliation may be sought when withdrawal of life-sustaining treatment is being considered, and an assurance can be given, not only for the comfort of the attending family, but also for nursing staff who have established a close bonding with the patient through many months of devoted care, that any possible discomfort associated with persisting awareness will be relieved by appropriate analgesia and/or sedation. If even only one family member suggests that the individual has preserved some awareness, it is reasonable to offer to administer sedation after hydration and nutrition are withdrawn. A subcutaneous infusion over 24 h using:

- *midazolam 5, 15 mg inj.; haloperidol 5 mg inj.* Midazolam 15–30 mg + haloperidol 5–15 mg or a bolus of phenobarbitone 200 mg daily should be effective for this purpose (see Section 4 PVS, p. 209).

SECTION IV

Ethical Issues

1

Consent and decision-making

Consent must be informed; it is a response to knowing the facts. Many of the facts in terminal illness are potentially sad and disturbing, but there is no justification for deliberately withholding information that will allow genuine informed consent.

The right to refuse treatment

In advanced neurological conditions there are a number of common situations in which continuation of life may depend on particular medical interventions. These include the performance of a gastrostomy to maintain nutrition in those unable to swallow, the provision of assisted ventilation for those whose respiratory function is severely impaired, or the treatment with antibiotics of an incidental infection (often respiratory).

In the judgement of some, if refusal of treatment leads to more rapid death, it ought not be allowed. In the opinion of others (including some governments), a patient can refuse medical treatment, but not the provision of food and drink if its refusal will lead to death, even if this is being administered by an 'artificial' route (intravenous (I-V), percutaneous endoscopic gastrostomy (PEG) and naso-gastric tube). This creates a distinction between nourishment and hydration on the one hand and the administration of drugs or surgery on the other. Still other persons and governments state that *any* patient has the right to refuse *any* medical intervention, even one that is regarded as the only way to sustain life.

The matter is made more complex by requiring a definition of 'medical treatment' or of 'artificial means'. Is feeding via a PEG or a naso-gastric tube a medical treatment; is a feeding tube 'artificial'? It has proved difficult to achieve consensus on such questions, though medical opinion is generally in favour of answering 'yes' to those questions (see section PVS below).

What if the patient is in no condition to indicate his or her wishes? Must those giving care assume that the actions required of them are those that sustain life? Sometimes family members will have strong feelings about what is right, but their requests may have no legal force. There can be no consistent response to that situation, and this is why the writing of advance directives and the appointment of surrogate decision-makers have been widely advocated.

2

Advance directives

The advance health care directive (or 'anticipatory direction') is an important component of the preparation by any individual for a time when some deterioration in individual competence is regarded as possible. It has been recommended as an important component of a routine medical examination at (say) the age of 75 years, or at the time of admission to an aged care facility. It becomes particularly relevant when the diagnosis of a potentially fatal condition has been made, and death and dying are a prospect requiring consideration. It provides an opportunity to clarify the range of possible outcomes and to indicate preferences for care. It can relieve family members and physicians of some of the burden of difficult decision-making.

An advance directive can rarely be both comprehensive and specific, because it is usually not possible to predict with any certainty the timing and nature of the final course of a terminal condition. Probably the most valuable aspect of raising the opportunity to write an advance directive is in the discussion that it arouses, and the permission that can follow to discuss difficult realities, and the options for facing them.

However, it may prove possible to indicate some particular wishes in response to the invitation: '*If you should become so ill that you are unable to speak for yourself, will you want to indicate the medical care you wish to receive?*'

For example, a patient may wish to indicate a desire to die at home, and state that only in circumstances that render adequate care too difficult for the family, should hospital admission be sought. A person suffering from amyotrophic lateral sclerosis (ALS) or muscular dystrophy may record that in the event of deterioration in respiratory function the emphasis of care must be on comfort rather than prolongation of life, and must not include tracheostomy. Or it may be decided to issue a clear direction not to be kept alive by artificial means of feeding or hydration.

A written advance directive may follow a form of words similar to this:

I [*full name and address*] direct that if, at some future time, I am in the terminal phase of an illness, or am regarded as being in a persistent vegetative state, effect is to be given to the following expression of my wishes (*then may follow one or more of the following*):

Please keep me comfortable and as free from pain as possible.

Do not transfer me to hospital unless absolutely necessary.

Request X-rays or blood tests only if the results will guide treatment to improve my comfort.

Prescribe antibiotics only if an infection is causing me discomfort.

I do not want life-sustaining treatment started. This includes cardiopulmonary resuscitation.

I do not want to receive artificial nutrition or hydration if they are treatments keeping me alive. If they have been started, I want them stopped.

[*Signed by person making the direction, and dated*]
[*Signed and dated by witness, and witness' full name and address*]

Such a document may also carry the provision that the directions may be rescinded or rewritten at any time while the writer remains competent.

Discussion carried out in preparation of an advance directive is generally regarded as promoting peace of mind and helping carers honour patient wishes; however, it could risk also the introduction of misunderstanding, coercion and promotion of either over-treatment or under-treatment, unless done with confidence that the person making the directive is fully informed.

3

Proxy decision-making

Cognition is compromised in many neurological conditions; often it is impossible to anticipate the onset of cognitive impairment. The timing and the extent of that impairment may be elusive, and the patient may worry that decisions regarding care will be made by individuals who have no awareness of his personality or priorities.

The patient may wish to designate a particular individual who is to be trusted to make decisions or give consent on the patient's behalf for medical or surgical treatments. Who is to take that responsibility? In some countries an individual patient can, while competent, formally appoint, by a duly witnessed, legally binding document, another person to be a medical advocate, a guardian and a surrogate decision-maker.

Where legislation to authorize the appointment of a proxy decision-maker is not in place, it may be possible to ensure that, during the earlier stages of an illness when cognition remains close to normal, matters of future directions are raised in ways that allow family members to feel confident about the patient's fears and hopes, and to know what are the patient's directions and wishes, in future times of potential difficulty. In such a case, a clear and agreed understanding among family members about 'what Mother said she wanted' can be very helpful, and guide compassionate medical care in the terminal stage. It may be taken into account if a legal judgment becomes necessary.

It is desirable that an advance directive or appointment of an agent be prepared with the full agreement of family members. However, at least some family members may wish that no such documents be prepared, or may want a form of words different from what the patient decides. In the setting of a family conference with members of the medical team, differences of perception and opinion can be shared, and the possibility of consensus explored.

The appointment of a Medical Agent may be written in these terms:

I [*full name and address*], appoint the following person(s) to be my medical agent(s) [*full names and addresses*] ....

I authorize my medical agent to make decisions about my medical treatment if I should become unable to do so for myself.

I require my medical agent to observe the following conditions and directions in exercising responsibility as my medical agent [*there may follow some provisions as in the writing of an advance directive*]

....

....

Witnessed by [*full name and address and signature*] on [*date*]

[There may be a list of the categories of persons able to act as witnesses, but the list will not include the treating physician or another medical colleague] The person(s) nominated as medical agent(s) must separately sign acceptance of the responsibility.

Family may be poorly informed about the illness and its stage; they may be denying the reality of deterioration and imminent death; they may feel guilty if participating in discussion about the time of dying or they may reject the discussion because they feel the patient is trying to save the family expense or prolonged responsibility for daily care.

The attending physician may be able to anticipate family tension, and seek to involve the important family members in the discussion before any words are framed for the document.

4

Ethical issues in states of disordered consciousness

Some situations of disordered consciousness present particular ethical challenges to families, professionals and society at large. In advanced neurological disease a patient may be unable to participate in decision-making; but there are potential treatment choices of great significance – to the level of a choice between life and death. Such situations demand the clearest possible clinical assessment (repeated over time when necessary), close and compassionate communication with attending family and staff, and a full awareness of the legal and cultural context within which care is being offered.

COMA

Coma is defined as a deep sustained pathological unconsciousness that results from dysfunction of the ascending reticular activating system in either the brainstem or both cerebral hemispheres. The patient cannot be aroused, and the eyes are closed. Coma may be transitory, or progress to persistent vegetative state (PVS) or brain death. Similarly, PVS may progress to coma.

PERSISTENT VEGETATIVE STATE (PVS)

The vegetative state is defined as a clinical condition of complete unawareness of the self and the environment, accompanied by sleep–wake cycles with either complete or partial preservation of hypothalamic and brainstem

Table IV.4.1   *Criteria for PVS*

Patients in a vegetative state show the following:

- No evidence of awareness of self or environment and an inability to interact with others.

- No evidence of sustained, reproducible, purposeful or voluntary behavioural responses to visual, auditory, tactile or noxious stimuli.

- No evidence of language comprehension or expression.

- Intermittent wakefulness manifested by the presence of sleep–wake cycles.

- Sufficiently preserved hypothalamic and brainstem autonomic functions to permit survival with medical and nursing care.

- Bowel and bladder incontinence.

- Variably preserved cranial nerve (pupillary, oculocephalic, corneal, vestibulo-ocular, gag) and spinal reflexes.

Practice parameters: Assessment and management of patients in the persistent vegetative state.
Quality Standards Subcommittee American Academy of Neurology. *Neurology* 1995; 45:1015–8.

autonomic functions. In Australia, a term preferred for PVS is 'Persistent Post-coma State', but this is not universally accepted (Table IV.4.1).

Such a vegetative state can be defined 'persistent' when it is present at one month after acute traumatic or non-traumatic brain injury, or is present for at least 1 month in degenerative or metabolic disorders or developmental malformations.

To use the term 'permanent vegetative state' implies an irreversible situation; this diagnosis, similarly, is not based on absolute criteria, but on probabilities; on a high degree of clinical certainty that the chance of regaining consciousness is exceedingly remote.

As Table IV.4.2 indicates, patients in a PVS show no signs of awareness or ability to respond to stimulus except in a reflex way. In this, they differ from those in a minimally conscious state (MCS) who demonstrate, though often inconsistently, appropriate responses to stimuli. These disturbances of consciousness are most likely to occur from severe head injury or cerebral anoxia (most often from cardiopulmonary arrest), but may also occur from degenerative or congenital nervous system disorders. PVS can be an outcome of Alzheimer's, Parkinson's, Creutzfeldt–Jabob or Huntington's diseases.

Table IV.4.2 *Comparison of clinical features associated with coma, PVS, MCS and LIS*

Condition	Consciousness	Sleep/ wake	Motor function	Auditory function	Visual function	Communication	Emotion
Coma	None	Absent	Reflex and postural responses only	None	None	None	None
PVS	None	Present	Postures or withdraws to noxious stimuli Occasional non-purposeful movement	Startle Brief orienting to sound	Startle Brief visual fixation	None	None Reflexive crying or smiling
MCS	Partial	Present	Localizes noxious stimuli Reaches for object Holds or touches objects in a manner that accommodates size and shape Automatic movements (e.g. scratching)	Localizes sound location Inconsistent command following	Sustained visual fixation Sustained visual pursuit	Contingent vocalization Inconsistent but intelligible verbalization or gesture	Contingent smiling or crying
LIS	Full	Present	Quadriplegic	Preserved	Preserved	Aphonic/ Anarthric Vertical eye movement and blinking usually intact	Preserved

LIS: locked-in syndrome.

Giacino JT, Ashwal S, Childs N, Cranford R, Jennet B, Katz DI, Kelly JP, Rosenberg JH, Whyte J, Zafonte RD, Zasler ND. The minimally conscious state. Definition and diagnostic criteria. *Neurology* 2002; 58:349–53.

MINIMALLY CONSCIOUS STATE (MCS)

MCS and PVS need to be distinguished, if possible, since in MCS there is greater chance of emerging into a higher state of consciousness; when consequent on acute traumatic brain injury up to 50% of patients diagnosed with MCS may achieve a state of moderate disability or better. As with PVS, however, the state may also be permanent, particularly where the cause has not been acute trauma.

The states of PVS and MCS occur because the brainstem resists hypoxia better than the higher cerebral centres, preserving the vegetative functions of pulse and respiration when centres subserving appreciation of stimuli and conscious expression have been inactivated, either temporarily or permanently. There is a spectrum of consequent outcomes, depending on which parts of the brain have been most involved, and extending from, on the one hand, brain death in which brainstem functions are also compromised, to, on the other hand, 'locked-in syndrome' (LIS) where there is recognizable continuing function of higher centres.

LOCKED-IN SYNDROME (LIS)

In LIS there is preservation of consciousness but an almost complete loss of ability to respond, only the movement of the eyes and blinking of the eyelids possibly being preserved. It is usually the result of limited damage to part of the brain; it may occur, for example, following brain trauma, in advanced multiple sclerosis (MS) or from a partial basilar artery thrombosis leading to a bilateral lesion of the ventral pons. The widespread availability of magnetic resonance imaging (MRI) now better alerts clinicians to the possibility of LIS by revealing a quite localized pontine lesion.

The preservation of eye movement gives a potential to communicate, but to appreciate that communication requires careful and intimate observation. Once recognized, it may be possible to establish a system of eye signals with the patient. The extent to which this can be successful is celebrated in the well-known text 'Le Scaphandre et le Papillon' (The Diving Bell and the Butterfly) written by Frenchman JD Bauby using only eye signals. Such an achievement took quite a long time, but there are many records of prolonged survival in this state. Recent developments in understanding the neural basis of language suggest that one day it may be possible to use electroencephalogram (EEG) information to 'read' words that form in consciousness, but no practical opportunity to do this can yet be envisaged. There are occasional reports of some functional recovery even months after the onset of

LIS, but in the great majority there will be further deterioration from additional vascular events or pulmonary complications leading to death.

LIS is, par excellence, a situation which demands intimate and very attentive nursing, not only to achieve good communication with well-phrased questions and comments that require only 'yes–no' answers, but also sensitive thoughtful handling of the patient in every respect: feeding to avoid aspiration (usually via a per-endoscopic gastrostomy PEG, also a route for medications); protecting the cornea and skin; moving and massaging the stiff limbs; medicating to relieve cramps and spasms and possibly central pain; caring for a urinary catheter. Most individuals will have a tracheostomy because of trouble caused by pharyngeal secretions and the risks of aspiration. Both depression (to which LIS patients are vulnerable, being unable to express their emotional pain and alienation) and problems with saliva will be assisted by regular amitriptyline; other antidepressants including selective serotonin reuptake inhibitors and mirtazepine may be preferred.

Restriction to very slow communication frustrates carers, who must be patient and tolerant when the individual with LIS is trying to spell out some important message. There is a temptation to jump in and finish the phrase for the patient, to respond in kind with brief messages (sometimes shouted, it will be difficult for some visitors to remember that the patient is fully alert and hears everything). The use of volunteers as well as family members, given some preparation and a willingness to sit and work quietly with the patient should be explored. Everyone working with the patient can learn the use of simple shorthand communication tools such as picture and alphabet boards. More sophisticated devices employ electronics, and can be made to respond to air pressure in the mouth, eyelid blinking or EEG. But any such complex machines will be useless without very careful and detailed preparation for both patient and those who will administer and maintain them.

Home care is possible only with a team of carers able to provide 24 h availability, and with routines in place that ensure that the patient can make needs known and be responded to promptly. If the major responsibility falls to a spouse or some other particular family member, that individual will need regular respite and comprehensive support.

This is not a situation calling for surrogate decision-makers (pp. 207–208), because the LIS patient ought to be able to make his or her own decisions clearly apparent. Decisions may involve matters of moving site of care, the use of mechanical ventilation or other treatment decisions. The most difficult issue may be an expressed desire to commit suicide when clearly there is no opportunity for the patient alone to effect it. There are only a few countries in which assisted suicide for such a patient would be countenanced and legally permissible, though many professional carers would see LIS as the setting within which they most would feel moved to provide such assistance in the face of a consistent request from the patient (see section on Euthanasia, p. 219).

THE MANAGEMENT OF PVS

In degenerative diseases, PVS of recent onset should alert the clinician to the possibility of some reversible element such as an acute infection or metabolic upset. Where PVS is persistent, superimposed infection is a common cause of death, and it will often be regarded as appropriate and ethical management to withhold specific treatment of the infection.

As there are reflex movements of eyes, face, limbs and even occasional vocalization family members will often interpret these as early signs of recovery, 'her eyes followed me around the bed'; 'she screwed up her face when her sister spoke to her'. Swallowing is no longer voluntary but food placed into the mouth may initiate a reflex swallowing action. A nasogastric tube or gastrostomy is usually necessary to maintain nutrition. To establish a diagnosis of PVS will usually require repeated careful observation over a period of some days, as there is no single clinical routine of examination which can confirm it with certainty.

As the causative event usually has been sudden and dramatic, vigorous and immediate efforts will have been made to maintain brain perfusion with assisted ventilation and cardiac support in an intensive care setting. There are no agreed interventions which will accelerate recovery, it is a matter of maintaining oxygenation and nutrition and waiting to see if any sign of consciousness returns. The longer a patient remains in this state, the less likely is any recovery. As weeks and months go by with no observable change, family and staff both need assistance to face the difficult reality that the individual on whom they have lavished so much careful attention may never improve. Occasional accounts of recovery after prolonged periods of vegetative state, however, give hope to families to wait and wait. Only a very small proportion of patients initially regarded as having PVS regain consciousness, but these cannot be predicted and the long-term outlook is not favourable.

The opinion of a neurologist should be sought to assist carers and family understand whether the state is 'permanent'. As a guide for carers and family, if there has been no evidence of any recovery after a period of 3 months following a non-traumatic brain injury or after 12 months following brain trauma, the state may be regarded as permanent. For the parents of small children in particular (such as toddlers rescued from drowning too late to avoid brain damage), this is a very stressful situation, and they are vulnerable to advice to engage in intense programmes of sensory stimulation and assisted movement, for the value of which there is still insufficient evidence.

The family as patient

While no interaction is possible with the PVS patient, much attention must be given to the attentive and anxious family members, who need to understand clearly the consequence of survival of brainstem function ('living') and the permanent damage ('death') to higher facilities of cerebral function. They can be reassured that there is no evidence of suffering, even though there may be occasional movements and grimaces.

The issue of making treatment decisions on behalf of the patient needs to be raised and clarified. Few individuals have made a clear statement of their wishes for management in advance of such a circumstance. One family member should assume responsibility for decision-making (in consultation with others if possible), and, in some countries, this can be given legal authority via application to a Guardianship Board or an equivalent legal body. Some important decisions will have been made in the early stages of the condition when the outcome was still quite uncertain: for example, the insertion of a urinary catheter, a tracheostomy or a gastrostomy, and these will have been guided largely by medical advice. Now, decisions may be required that depend less on medical advice. For example, a further site of care: home, nursing home or hospice; whether to continue active treatment of recurrent infection (e.g. of the chest); or whether to withdraw nutritional support and focus on ensuring, as far as possible, a comfortable death. PVS patients almost certainly do not experience pain, but if there are reflex responses to some stimuli, it should be acceptable to give a continuous subcutaneous (S/C) infusion of opioid and sedative, and this will usually be immensely reassuring for family members. A decision to withdraw nutritional support can be interpreted, in discussions with family, as in no way a discounting of the importance and value of the affected individual, but as an expression of love and compassion.

The terminal phase

Given attentive management and prompt treatment for urinary and chest infection, some persons with PVS may continue in that state for years. Home care is enormously demanding if it is to be open ended in duration.

The 'terminal phase' may therefore only be established when a decision to withhold treatment for an infection or to withdraw nutritional support has been reached. A family may elect to take the patient home to die, and to accept the role of surrounding the patient with their loving presence and support for the few days that remain after withdrawal of tubes and nutrition. Such home care can be a rich experience for family members; sad, but welcomed as the best possible outcome.

Provision and withdrawal of nutritional support in PVS

Whether it is acceptable to withdraw nutritional support that is maintaining the PVS state is determined by cultural and religious factors, medical tradition, law and established precedent. The question of to what extent a person in PVS ought be regarded as 'alive' or already 'dead' is not assisted by knowledge of the variety of neurological, religious and legal pronouncements that have sought to address this situation. Increasingly, however, the wish of family to cease life support, and the willingness of professional attendants to agree with, for example, withdrawal of nutritional support, is being given weight in a number of countries, and may become more widely accepted as legitimate and humane practice. In its decision in the case of Nancy Cruzan, the US Supreme Court affirmed that all US citizens may refuse any medical treatment, including treatment regarded as life-sustaining, and even the provision of artificial means of nutrition and hydration. They also ruled that a surrogate person may exercise this right on behalf of an incompetent individual.

In 1988, the American Academy of Neurology released a statement on *the Care and Management of the Persistent Vegetative State Patient*. The statement includes these paragraphs:

> 'The artificial provision of nutrition and hydration is a form of medical treatment and may be discontinued in accordance with the principles and practices governing the withholding and withdrawal of other forms of medical treatment.'
>
> 'The administration of fluids and nutrition by medical means, such as a gastric tube, is a medical procedure rather than a nursing procedure.'
>
> 'When a patient has been reliably diagnosed as being in a persistent vegetative state, and when it is clear that the patient would not want further medical treatment, and the family agrees with the patient, all further medical treatment, including the artificial provision of nutrition and hydration, may be foregone.'

Contrary opinion may be forcefully expressed, as in the widely publicized case of Terri Schiavo in the US in 2005. Here, the argument in favour of maintaining nutrition via a feeding tube related primarily to a religious affirmation of the sanctity of human life and that Terri's life was still to be valued and respected after 15 years of PVS:

> 'Our God is in the business of protecting and nourishing broken, discarded lives which seem to have little meaning. He can use these tragedies to let his glory shine into a dark and painful world. His images should respond likewise'.
>
> *Donal P. O'Mathuna. Philosophia Christi 1996; 19(2 Fall):55–83.*

There is also a common claim that to withdraw feeding condemns such a patient to a 'horrible death', a period of suffering through starvation and dehydration. Palliative care experience suggests that withdrawal of nutrition in such situations results in no discernible suffering, but if it is necessary to reassure family members about this, a continuous S/C infusion of opioid and sedation can be provided.

A more objective and evidence-based approach is found in the document 'Practice Parameters: Assessment and Management of Patients in the Persistent Vegetative State', prepared by the American Academy of Neurology (see Suggested further reading).

Terminal sedation

There is little doubt that the provision of continuous analgesia and sedation to reduce discomfort in the terminal phase of any illness can hasten death, if only by a matter of hours, though usually not in any rapid or predictable timescale.

Families who have stayed patiently by the side of a slowly deteriorating patient with a terminal illness commonly welcome the release and the relief that follows the final onset of death. But they can easily worry that by assenting to an offer of sedation, they have been complicit in a form of euthanasia.

They will need time to ask questions and hear staff responses. It will be suggested that there is no intention to kill in providing this therapy; the aim is to ensure that dying (which is happening anyway) is free from any distress of pain, restlessness or delirium. What is being provided is a continuing appropriate treatment for the patient, not some new and different intervention carrying a potentially illegal and fatal consequence.

Some families will ask that sedation and analgesia be withheld. They may hold a hope that the patient has some communication to make in the dying moments (an expectation possibly fostered by the depiction of death on television) or they may have religious objections to sedation at this time. Some Buddhist traditions, for example, hope for full lucidity and awareness at the moment of death as an important component of satisfactory reincarnation.

In most western traditions, however, families and staff will find it acceptable and helpful to ensure that the immediate dying phase is free from any pain and suffering, and a continuation of the infusion of an opioid and benzodiazepine (morphine, hydromorphone, fentanyl or diamorphine plus midazolam or clonazepam) will be welcomed.

Euthanasia

There can be no doubt that the terminal phase of many neurological diseases may involve serious suffering (physical, emotional and spiritual). Although such situations are often endured with exemplary courage and patience, they also inevitably raise questions of the value of continued life in the face of persistent suffering, or permanent incapacity for effective cognition or movement. Is a hastening of the process of dying to be preferred? A hierarchy of options for hastening death to relieve severe suffering may be listed. Some are more acceptable to public opinion than others; some are more readily countenanced by established medical ethics; some are advocated widely but allowed in very few countries.

(a) *Allowing the patient to refuse all food and drink.* A conscious patient in most jurisdictions is permitted to refuse treatment, and in some places may also be permitted to refuse nutrition, and be assisted to remain comfortable through a period of terminal decline (often referred to as 'starvation', but this is an emotive term, better kept for an imposed restriction of food rather than one which is self-chosen). A demented patient may be difficult to feed, clamping the mouth shut, turning the head away. Some clinicians suggest that such individuals should not be forced to receive nutrition (e.g. with a nasogastric tube) but permitted to refrain from food and drink as they seem to wish. In other situations, however, this is expressly forbidden (either by established medical ethic or by law) and physicians are required to maintain nutrition in some way.

(b) *Refraining from potentially life-sustaining treatment, or ceasing it.* Such treatment may include antibiotic therapy, tube feeding or assisted ventilation. It is recognized that, in most instances where there is doubt about the value of such measures, it is more difficult to cease them than to refrain from starting them. After tube feeding has commenced, its withdrawal will appear to some observers the removal of an artificial, intrusive and unnecessary intervention, but to others will be a deliberate act of killing. (The example mentioned earlier of Terri Schiavo, whose death in March 2005 followed withdrawal of a feeding tube after 15 years in an apparent vegetative state, illustrated the polarization of opinion that may accompany such an action.)

Difference of opinion is likely to be seen most clearly in the removal of life-sustaining assisted ventilation via tracheostomy, when death may follow very soon after its withdrawal. In some jurisdictions the law forbids that removal absolutely, in which case it may be felt that it would be better not to start it.

(c) *Intensive symptom management that may shorten life*. Sometimes, to overcome severe pain, analgesia needs to be increased to the extent that the patient is barely responsive. In such situations, discussion often centres on *intention*, or on '*double effect*'. It may be seen as acceptable to treat with high doses of opioid if the intention is to relieve pain; death then coming as a secondary effect, not the primary effect sought. But it would be regarded as unacceptable to give the same medication if the intention was to deliberately shorten life. Physicians are therefore required to communicate openly their plan of treatment and the intention of the medication regimen that is being implemented.

(d) *Heavy sedation to relieve intractable symptoms not otherwise controlled*. Where either physical or emotional discomfort is otherwise difficult to overcome, it may be possible to induce a state of sleep or an unconscious state with continuous sedation, allowing the patient to remain so through to the time of death. Such a course may be labelled 'slow-stream euthanasia' by some; sensible symptom palliation by others. Here again, there is a issue of *intention* and a need for transparent and open communication of the medical plan of treatment.

(e) *Assisting death at the patient's request (physician-assisted suicide)*. This may occur for a conscious and active patient by prescribing medication that the patient can self-administer (a large oral dose of barbiturate) or it may entail administration of a fatal dose of medication (e.g. I-V barbiturate with potassium) by the physician. The former is what has been permitted in Oregon (USA), the latter is permitted in the Netherlands. Such actions have been strongly condemned by palliative care services.

Legislation to permit physician-assisted suicide has usually required that:

- the patient be judged to have a *terminal illness*;
- there be judged to be *intolerable suffering*;
- the option of effective symptom control (or palliative care advice and opinion) has been provided and found unsatisfactory;
- a second medical opinion of the terminal nature of the disease and the condition of the patient has been obtained;
- a waiting period elapses before euthanasia may proceed.

Requests to hasten death may come from the patient, but in neurological illness may also be raised by relatives, because the patient is lacking either cognitive or expressive capacity. In Oregon (USA), where physician-assisted suicide has been possible since 1999, 8% of a total of 208 individuals who have taken this course were suffering from ALS; 2.5% from human immunodeficiency virus(HIV)/acquired immune deficiency syndrome (AIDS); 79% had malignant neoplasms. As even close relatives may have their own reasons (sometimes compassionate and altruistic, sometimes personal and self-serving) for recommending a shortening of the dying period, it is helpful to attending physicians if the patient has been able to make a relevant advanced directive, or has appointed an alternate medical decision-maker with a legally valid document.

A strong advocacy in support of euthanasia is established in many Western countries. It promotes the preparation of legislation to allow patients to access physician-assistance in having death hastened deliberately. This presents considerable difficulty, as indicated by the need to define '*terminal illness*' and '*intolerable suffering*' in the above list of requirements. The factors driving advocacy are partly cultural, drawing on the primacy in the West of considerations of individual autonomy; partly demographic and economic, taking note of the increased numbers of very aged receiving expensive but less than adequate care in growing numbers of institutions; partly a desire to avoid a medicalized death at the hands of an arrogant medical profession.

There are also religious attitudes contributing to the debate, affirming the sacred and inviolable quality of life and resisting any action that might shorten it, along with more liberal religious opinion promoting a loving response to the perceived dying wish of the suffering individual, whatever request is made.

The issue remains contentious, but debate is certain to continue. Greater use of the opportunity to write advanced directive and medical power of attorney instructions may help broaden experience and encourage greater consensus within communities where no agreement has existed.

In the Netherlands, since 2002, physician-assisted suicide has been allowed for a patient with 'unbearable and incurable' suffering. Examples of assisted suicide have been reported recently from that country in cases of Alzheimer's disease (one case) and Huntington's disease (three cases). In these instances, the assistance was provided before the disease had reached a phase when the patient could be regarded as terminally ill; these individuals considered themselves unable to face the prospect of the suffering ahead, and chose to end life before that stage was reached.

SECTION V

Appendices

1

Practical aspects of home care

NECESSARY SUPPORTS

Satisfactory care at home for an individual with an advanced or terminal neurological condition will usually require, or benefit from:

1. *24-h availability of a competent carer*: In modern family structures, it is not uncommon for individuals to live alone. For the care of an individual with advanced neurological disease it will usually be necessary for there to be an effective carer available at all times. If funding allows, this need may be met by a round-the-clock roster of nurses or paramedical staff; more often it will depend on the availability of family members.
2. *A suitable home environment*: This may need to allow accessibility by a wheelchair from outside, and free movement within the dwelling on one level, availability of private and quiet space, opportunity to install special equipment (e.g. railings, a hospital bed) and suitable bathroom and toilet facilities.
3. *Regular availability of dependable visiting support services*; for example community nurses, family medical practitioners able to undertake house calls, equipment services.
4. *Availability of 24-h specialist telephone advice* from a member of a team familiar with the patient's situation, who is able to access basic records and is knowledgeable about palliation measures.

These requirements will frequently not be available. Many homes are hardly suitable for satisfactory home care of advanced disease. They are too small, or too cluttered with necessary furnishings to accept helpful equipment (even if it was available). Some will be in a high-rise building and not served by an elevator. There is often no one person or roster of persons able to be present at all times to maintain care; no visiting nurse service that can be afforded, no family doctor willing to visit on a regular basis, no physician or specialist nurse or telephone service able to listen to problems and offer advice on a 24-h basis.

THE HOME ENVIRONMENT

If home care is preferred, there are many environmental components to be considered:

1. If the patient is confined to bed, the best site for the bed may be in a room where friends and relatives can readily visit; it may look onto an outside area, on a small garden. If it is possible to bring in a hospital bed, with electrical power for altering height and lifting either end, nursing care will be much facilitated. Attachments to assist mobility may be useful for some patients – overhead grip, bedside rails. There needs to be some way for the patient to call for assistance – a bell able to be activated with minimal effort, for instance. Objects that the patient may be able to use – tissues, a drinking cup, a telephone, should be able to be easily reached on a table by the bed.

   Familiar objects comforting to the patient should be in the room – pictures, photographs, flowers, a radio, favourite objects (e.g. a vase, a clock).

2. If the patient is able to spend part of the day out of bed, a comfortable chair needs to be placed in a good spot, perhaps one with an outside view, good lighting, handy to toilet and bathroom.

3. If the patient is weak in standing, the toilet seat may need to be raised, and rails fitted to assist seating and standing.

4. There should be a small chair for visitors to use beside the bed.

5. A bathroom may be difficult for a dependent patient to use. A plastic chair that can be placed in a shower recess or near the drain hole in the floor will allow the use of a shower hose.

6. Medications for the patient need to be kept safe in a high cupboard out of the reach of children, and carefully labelled so that dose and time of administration is well recognized.

7. The patient may be able to move outside only with assistance, perhaps with a walking frame or in a wheelchair. Doors may need to be changed to open outwards rather than into a room, ramps may need to be installed to allow movement into the garden area.

Equipment to be considered

- Ramps at home entrances
- Hospital bed
- Bed stick (a small pole facilitating moving in and out of bed)
- Toilet raiser
- Commode
- Shower chair
- Lifter
- Mattress overlay (sheepskin, eggshell foam, air mattress)
- Wheelchair

EDUCATION FOR HOME CARERS

Many family members will have had little or no nursing experience. Preparation for what will often be a long and onerous commitment should include advice and demonstration for:

- lifting and transferring a patient with impaired mobility;
- showering the patient or washing the patient in bed;
- management of bladder and bowels;
- regular recording of medication usage;
- assessment and reporting of changes in the patient's condition;
- administration of medication (by mouth, per-endoscopic gastrostomy (PEG) or intermittent injection);
- maintenance of a subcutaneous infusion;
- managing visits and offers of assistance by friends and relatives;
- looking after yourself – ensuring respite periods and effective sleep.

COMMON QUESTIONS RAISED BY HOME CARERS

What will happen next?
Often not easy to answer, but the carers may be reassured by knowing that any change can be reported and will receive serious consideration and prompt response.

How long do we have?
The uncertainty of prognosis must be conveyed. Estimates will often be inaccurate. As the terminal phase progresses, it will become more possible to make appropriate estimates of the probable time of death.

How will death happen? What will it be like?
It is sometimes quite difficult to anticipate the mode of death. Although the continuation of a process of deterioration that has been under observation is most likely, new complications (e.g. a pulmonary embolus) may supervene. Most likely death will be a quiet, slow change in consciousness, respiration and pulse, with no dramatic event.

How will I know that death is approaching, or has occurred?
A change in respiration, with periods of apnoea and deep breaths, a cooling of the extremities, a weakening of the pulse and a failure of any response are common signs that death is near. A cool body with no evidence of respiration will usually be recognizable. Make sure that the carers know how to access a person competent to confirm death.

If care becomes too difficult at home, where can we get help?
This is a critical component of a coordinated care plan (pp. 20–21). Home carers should know in advance and have confidence that nurse or medical re-assessment can be accessed to review the home situation and suggest alternatives, if necessary.

ADVANTAGES OF HOME CARE

1. Immediate care is available throughout 24 h. In hospital or other care institutions, nursing staff can offer only limited time for the care of any individual; at home, a family member is usually present at all times.
2. Familiar surroundings offer a greater opportunity to relax; a greater sense of control in situations where, in hospital, the patient may feel dependent, lacking a voice in what is decided for care.
3. Easy access for other family members and friends. This may need monitoring, so that the patient is not exhausted by trying to be responsive. Friends may need to be told to limit stays to no more than a few minutes.

THE IMPORTANCE OF A RECORD IN THE HOME

Carers should be encouraged to maintain a record of the patient's care which might include:

1. A day-by-day record of simple observations about the patient's condition – mobility, alert or drowsy, lucid or confused, any pain,

nausea, urine output, bowel action, communicating or not, diet and fluid intake.

2. An account of each medication prescribed and taken – dose, time administered, plus any comment on useful or untoward effect.

3. Space for comments by visiting professionals, who should be encouraged to use the record to coordinate their individual contributions.

2

Characteristics of an effective palliation service

AN ACCEPTED PLACE IN NATIONAL HEALTH PLANNING

In many countries, the recognition of palliation as an integral part of the national health effort has been minimal, or slow to develop. Without strong advocacy from within the general community or the health professions there has been little action on the part of government to provide legislation, regulation or funding to support palliation delivery.

Legislation can assist by any one of the following:

- Requiring patient consent for both the provision and the withdrawal of medical treatment.
- Authorizing the opportunity to write advance directives for future care.
- Authorizing the appointment of a medical agent to make decisions on behalf of an incompetent patient.

Government regulation will be required to allow the following:

- The ready prescription of palliation medications (e.g. opioids) in community as well as hospital settings.
- Subsidizing the availability of palliation medications to the needy.
- Funding for community care resources to support home care. This may be through extension of health insurance to cover community care or through a specific allocation for funding home care within the health budget.
- The inspection and accreditation of care institutions (including chronic care and aged care facilities) to maintain standards in the provision of palliation.
- A designated section within the health bureaucracy to support palliation care in both cancer and non-cancer diseases.

Government funding of public in-patient facilities should allow a focus on palliation through the establishment of designated staff positions (medical, nursing and allied health), and the remuneration of palliation activities in private institutions by insurance providers should be adequate to encourage this type of care.

Palliation needs recognition as a clinical responsibility within medicine generally, and to that end requires the establishment of undergraduate and postgraduate education programs to help all relevant specialities improve their capacity to provide effective palliation.

PALLIATION SERVICES ARE ORGANIZED ON A POPULATION BASIS

For the *advanced neurological diseases* that are the major interest of this publication, the usual focus on neurology teams based in large hospitals should be supplemented by a close link with care provided in home sites and chronic care facilities. It is possible for many individuals with these diseases to receive much of their terminal care at home, and home nursing services are a critical component of the necessary palliation resources. This will be achieved if there are between 30 and 70 nurses with a specialist responsibility for palliation in each population of 1 million persons, supported by multidisciplinary neurological teams who accept responsibility for the community oversight of home care as well as hospital admissions. If generalist community nurses are available in greater numbers to oversee all types of home care, a small number (10–15) of specialist palliation nurse providers may be sufficient to supervise, advise and educate the generalist nurses who undertake most of the daily home nursing duty.

It is also desirable that specialist palliative care teams be available to offer expert opinion and support for particular cases, whether in large hospital, home, and aged care or chronic disease facility.

PALLIATION TEAMS ARE ESTABLISHED AND MAINTAINED

The work of delivering palliation care typically attracts individuals who enjoy the challenge of engaging with patients and families in potentially sad and uncomfortable circumstances. They share with patients and family members the disappointments of failed therapies, they recognize the incipient grief being experienced, they evince a compassion and a dedication that is compelling. But the needs of their patients are often huge and continuous, and no one individual can meet those needs. Effective teamwork is an essential component of palliation practice, requiring good communication and handing over of responsibility within each participating professional group, but also a flexibility and a mutual respect across the usual professional barriers that separate nurse and doctor, for example. Volunteers are also valued members of such a team, providing practical relief for families through 'time-out' sitting with the patient at home to allow the carer to shop or visit, sometimes providing simple complementary measures such as hand or foot massage or aromatherapy, and always offering companionship and interest to an individual whose world has shrunk to the confines of a bed.

It is desirable that patients and their supporting family members be given clear information about whom they can contact, and how. The contact numbers of all, or at least some team members will be very reassuring. At the same time, the agreed goals of the team's work together should be recorded so that all are reminded of their shared commitment.

The model of care being proposed is subversive, in that it refuses to recognize some of the boundaries within health care that have formerly separated hospital from home, doctor from nurse, specialist from generalist, modern medicine from traditional and alternative practice.

EDUCATION FOR PALLIATION IS ESTABLISHED

In introducing a recent text on Palliative Care and Neurology, Dr Kathleen Foley wrote: 'Increasing appreciation of the importance of palliative care for patients with neurological disorders has been emphasized by the Ethics and Humanities Committee of the American Academy of Neurology in its 1996 position statement which said: "*It is imperative: ... that neurologists understand and learn to apply the principles of palliative care as ... many patients with neurologic disease die after long illnesses during which the neurologist acts as principal or consulting physician.*"'

The preparation of a neurologist for future practice must encourage familiarity not only with the traditional careful clinical neurological examination and its interpretation in the light of sophisticated investigations, but also the many new developments that promise effective interventions for diseases previously inaccessible to modification. At the same time, however, it will be increasingly apparent that the burden of progressive degenerative disease continues to increase, and it will require that the modern neurologist be a focus of advice and expertise not only in measures founded in stem-cell, genetic and surgical modification of disease, but also in basic care and symptom control for the many thousands who will continue to face a sad and uncomfortable decline.

In several countries, palliative care has won recognition as a medical speciality, and is established with its own postgraduate training programme. So far, the emphasis has been on cancer, with placements in oncology or radiotherapy services required as well as an extended period in a palliative care inpatient setting. Training could be much broader in scope, and build on training and experience in other specialities: neurology, psychiatry, geriatrics, pain management, family practice are appropriate. In those countries where the speciality of palliative care is established, it will be some 5 years after completion of an undergraduate course that a physician achieves speciality status in palliative medicine.

Modules for teaching palliation can be incorporated into any specialist training, (including neurology), and can also be made available for family practitioners, nurses and other professional categories.

As currently established, specialist palliative care providers can attend to only a small proportion of those who die in any community, their role will be to focus on the more difficult cases (still mainly advanced cancer), and on the support and education of other health staff who are undertaking the greater part of care for individuals with advanced and terminal illness, including the progressive neurological diseases.

Undergraduate courses in medicine, nursing and ancillary health professions should provide an introduction to basic palliation. Further, the preparation of a wide range of specialists should also incorporate both theoretical and practical exposure to symptom management in all its dimensions.

3

Suggested further reading

GENERAL TEXTS

Addington-Hall J, Higginson I (eds). *Palliative Care for Non-cancer Patients*. OUP, Oxford, 2001.
[Considers the care needs and service provision for a wide range of patients with terminal disease due to non-cancer conditions, including neurodegenerative disease, stroke and dementia.]

Ahmedzai SH, Muers MF (eds). *Supportive Care in Respiratory Disease*. OUP, Oxford, 2005.
[A recent publication that highlights the value of a palliation approach to management of another specialty area.]

Carver AC, Foley KM (eds). *Palliative Care. Neurologic Clinics* 2001; 19(4): 789–1044, published by WB Saunders, Philadelphia.
[A more selective text, addressing care for ALS, Huntington's, dementia, brain tumours and stroke, with reference to general management and ethical issues.]

Doyle D, Hanks GWC, Macdonald N (eds). *Oxford Textbook of Palliative Medicine*. OUP, Oxford, 1999.
[A comprehensive and authoritative reference for the management of terminal illness, but with a particular emphasis on advanced cancer.]

Kite S, O'Doherty C. *Palliative care*. In: Raj GS, Mulley GP (eds). *Elderly Medicine: A Training Guide*. Cambridge University Press, Cambridge, 2002.
[Discusses the palliative care approach to meeting the needs of the geriatric population.]

Samuels MA (ed.). *Manual of Neurologic Therapeutics*, 7th edition. Lippincott Williams & Wilkins, Philadelphia, 2004.
[A didactic tightly-packed pocket book detailing management of neurological diseases, likely to prove of value to non-neurologists who wish to know what has gone before in the experience of individuals approach end-of-life care.]

Voltz R, Bernat JL, Borasio GD, Maddocks I, Oliver D, Portney RK (eds). *Palliative Care in Neurology*. OUP, Oxford, 2004.
[The first comprehensive text addressing end-of-life care for major degenerative neurological diseases.]

Watson M, Lucas C, Hoy A, Back I. *Oxford Handbook of Palliative Care*. OUP, Oxford, 2005.

[Based on the larger *Oxford Textbook of Palliative Medicine*, this text provides summaries covering practical advice on symptom management, again emphasizing cancer care.]

WEB SITES

There is a proliferation of web sites providing both authoritative and alternative information on all aspects of neurological conditions. Those listed below link to credible national organizations established to assist individuals affected by these conditions and also their family members, briefly indicating aspects of diagnosis, investigation, treatment and the availability of information and support service:

Multiple sclerosis
USA: www.nmss.org
UK: www.mssociety.org.uk
Canada: www.mssociety.ca
Australia: www.msaustralia.org.au

Amyotrophic lateral sclerosis (motor neurone disease)
USA: www.alsa.org
Canada: www.als.ca
UK: www.mndassociation.org
Australia: www.mnd.asn.au
New Zealand: www.mndanz.org.nz

Dementia
UK: www.alzheimers.org.uk
USA: www.alz.org
Canada: www.alzheimer.ca

Parkinson's disease
World: www.wpda.org
USA: www.pdf.org
UK: www.parkinsons.org.uk
Europe: www.epda.eu.com
Australia: www.parkinsons.org.au

Huntington's disease
USA: www.hdsa.org
UK: www.hda.org.uk
Australia: www.ahda.asn.au
Canada: www.hsc-ca.org

Muscular dystrophy

>Australia: www.mda.org.au
>Canada: www.mdac.ca

Brain trauma and stroke

>http://www.braintrauma.org
>http://www.strokefoundation.com.au/
>www.stroke.org

Euthanasia

>news.bbc.co.uk/hi/english/static/health/euthanasia/basics.stm
>[*BBC site offering objective summaries of different approaches to this controversial issue.*]
>http://www.nvve.nl/english
>[*Provides text of the Netherlands law allowing physician-assisted suicide.*]
>http://www.dwd.org/law/ohd.asp
>[*Links to Oregon's Death with Dignity legislation and provides statistics of those availing themselves of this legislation.*]

Creutzfeldt–Jakob disease (CJD)

>www.fortunecity.com/healthclub/cpr/798/cjd.htm
>[*Stories from family members of patients who died from CJD.*]

JOURNAL ARTICLES

These have been drawn mainly from recent literature and are selective, aimed at listing relevant contributions to palliative management for neurological disorders that have appeared in either the neurology journals or in major palliative care journals. There are not so many, and many of the headings in this book are not represented in this literature.

Introduction
Recording of symptoms

Bruera E, Kuehn N, Miller MJ, Selmser P, Macmillian K. The Edmonton symptom assessment system (ESAS) a simple method for the assessment of palliative care patients. *Journal of Palliative Care* 1991; 7(2): 6–9.

Spiritual issues

Strang P, Strang S, Hultborn R, Arner S. Existential pain – an entity, a provocation, or a challenge? *Journal of Pain and Symptom Management* 2004; 27(3): 241–50.

Symptom management
Fatigue

Chaudhuri A, Behan PO. Fatigue in neurological disorders. *Lancet* 2004; 363: 978–88.

Spasticity, muscle cramps

Chou R, Peterson K, Helfand M. Comparative efficacy and safety of skeletal muscle relaxants for spasticity and musculoskeletal conditions: a systematic review. *Journal of Pain and Symptom Management* 2004; 28(2): 140–75.

Snow BJ, Tsui JK, Bhatt MH, Varelas M, Hashimoto SA, Calne DB. Treatment of spasticity with botulinum toxin: a double-blind study. *Annals of Neurology* 1990; 28: 512–15.

Young RR. Spasticity: a review. *Neurology* 1994; 44(Suppl. 9): S12–20.

Dysphagia

Kirker FJ, Oliver DJ. The development and implementation of a standardized policy for the management of dysphagia in motor neurone disease. *Palliative Medicine* 2003; 17(4): 322–6.

Drooling

Lucas V, Ammass C. The use of oral glycopyrrolate in drooling (Letter). *Palliative Medicine* 1998; 12: 207.

Ventilator issues

Kaub-Wittemer D, Steinbuchel N, Wasner M, Laier-Groeneveld G, Borasio GD. Quality of life and psychosocial issues in ventilated patients with amyotrophic lateral sclerosis and their caregivers. *Journal of Pain and Symptom Management* 2003; 26(4): 890–6.

Death rattle

Back IN, Jenkins K, Blower A, Beckhelling J. A study comparing hyoscine hydrobromide and glycopyrrolate in the treatment of death rattle. *Palliative Medicine* 2001; 15(4): 329–36.

Kass RM, Ellershaw J. Respiratory tract secretions in the dying patient: a retrospective study. *Journal of Pain and Symptom Management* 2003; 26(4): 897–902.

Wildiers H, Menten J. Death rattle: prevalence, prevention and treatment. *Journal of Pain and Symptom Management* 2002; 23(4): 310–17.

Neuropathic pain

Chong MS, Bajwa ZH. Diagnosis and treatment of neuropathic pain. *Journal of Pain and Symptom Management* 2003; 25(Suppl. 5): S4–11.

Dworkin RH, Backonja M, Rowbotham MC, *et al.* Advances in neuropathic pain. *Archives of Neurology* 2003; 60: 1524–34.

Kannan TR, Saxena A, Bhatnagar S, Barry A. Oral ketamine as an adjuvant to oral morphine for neuropathic pain in cancer patients. *Journal of Pain and Symptom Management* 2002; 2: 60–5.

Central pain

Leijon G, Boivie J, Johansson I. Central post-stroke pain – neurological symptoms and pain characteristics. *Pain* 1989; 36(1): 13–25.

Other strategies for difficult pain: ketamine

Fitzgibbon EJ, Hall P, Schroder C, Seely J, Viola R. Low dose ketamine as an analgesic adjuvant in difficult pain syndromes: a strategy for conversion from parenteral to oral ketamine. *Journal of Pain and Symptom Management* 2002; 23(2): 165–70.

Urological symptoms

Mattson D, Petrie M, Srivastava DK, McDermott M. Multiple sclerosis. Sexual dysfunction and its response to medications. *Archives of Neurology* 1995; 52: 862–8.

Delirium

Fainsinger RL. Treatment of delirium at the end of life: medical and ethical issues. In: Portnoy RK, Briera E (eds). *Topics in Palliative Care*, Vol. 4. OUP, Oxford, 2000.

Agitation, restlessness

Alexopoulos GS, Silver JM, Kahn DA, Frances A, Carpenter D (eds). *The Expert Consensus Guideline Series: Agitation in Older Persons with Dementia*. A Postgraduate Medicine Special Report. McGraw Hill April, 1998. www.psychguides.com/gagl/pdf

Brodaty H, Ames D, Snowdon J, Woodward M, Kirwan J, Clarnette R, Lee E, Lyons B, Grossman F. A randomized placebo-controlled trial of risperidone for the treatment of aggression, agitation, and psychosis of dementia. *Journal of Clinical Psychiatry* 2003; 64(2): 134–43.

Grief and bereavement

Chochinov H, Katz L. Abnormal bereavement: diagnosis, management, and prevention. In: Portnoy RK, Briera E (eds). *Topics in Palliative Care*, Vol. 2. OUP, Oxford, 2000.

Major neurological conditions

Cerebrovascular diseases and stroke

Widar M, Ek AC, Ahlstrom G. Coping with long-term pain after a stroke. *Journal of Pain and Symptom Management* 2004; 27(3): 215–25.

Demyelinating diseases (multiple sclerosis (MS) and acute demyelinating encephalomyelitis (ADEM))

Goodin DS. Survey of multiple sclerosis in northern California. Northern California MS Study Group. *Multiple Sclerosis* 1999; 5: 78–88.

Moulin DE, Foley KM, Ebers GC. Pain syndromes in multiple sclerosis. *Neurology* 1988; 38: 1830–4.

Svendsen KB, Jensen TS, Overvad K, *et al.* Pain in patients with multiple sclerosis. *Archives of Neurology* 2003; 60: 1089–94.

Parkinson's disease and related disorders (striato-nigral degeneration (SND), cortico-basilar degeneration (CBD), multiple system atrophy (MSA) and progressive supranuclear palsy (PSP))

Schrag A, Ben-Shlomo Y, Quinn N. How common are complications of Parkinson's disease? *Journal of Neurology* 2002; 249(4): 419–23.

Dementia

Abbey J, Piller N, de Bellis A, Estermann A, Parker D, Giles L, Lowcay B. The Abbey pain scale: a 1 minute numerical indicator for people with end stage dementia. *International Journal of Palliative Nursing* 2004; 10(1): 6–13.

Manfredi PL, Breuer B, Meier DE, Libow L. Pain assessment in elderly patients with severe dementia. *Journal of Pain and Symptom Management* 2003; 25(1): 48–52.

The American Academy of Family Physicians. <familydoctor.org/585.xml> [Practical advice for families living with a person suffering from dementia.]

Zeisel J, Silverstein NM, Hyde J, Levkoff S, Lawton MP, Holmes W. Environmental correlates to behavioral health outcomes in Alzheimer's special care units. *Gerontologist* 2003; 43: 697–711.

Amyotrophic lateral sclerosis, ALS (motor neurone disease)

Ganzini L, Silveira MJ, Johnston WS. Predictors and correlates of interest in assisted suicide in the final month of life among ALS patients in Oregon and Washington. *Journal of Pain and Symptom Management* 2002; 24(3): 312–17.

Hecht MJ, Graesel E, Tigges S, Hillemacher T, Winterholler M, Hilz MJ, Heuss D, Neundorfer B. Burden of care in amyotrophic lateral sclerosis. *Palliative Medicine* 2003; 17(4): 327–33.

Oliver D, Borasio GD, Walsh D (eds). *Palliative Care in Amyotrophic Lateral Sclerosis.* Oxford University Press, Oxford, 2000.

University of Montana Practical Ethics Centre: *Completing the Continuum of ALS Care: A Consensus Document.* Workgroup Recommendations to the Field. [Available on-line from www.promotingexcellence.org]

Welling Anne D. *Amyotrophic Lateral Sclerosis: Lou Gehrig's Disease.* http://www.aafp.org/afp/990315ap/1489.html

Viral and prion infections (human immunodeficiency virus (HIV) and CJD)

Brandel JP, Delasnerie-Lauprêtre N, Laplanche JL, Hauw JJ, Alpérovitch A. Diagnosis of Creutzfeldt–Jakob disease: effect of clinical criteria on incidence estimates. *Neurology* 2000; 54: 1095–9.

Brew BJ. *HIV Neurology. Contemporary Neurology Series.* OUP, Oxford, 2001.

University of Montana Practical Ethics Centre: *HIV Care: An Agenda for Change.* Workgroup Recommendations to the Field. [Available on-line from www.promotingexcellence.org]

Huntington's disease

Rosenblatt A, Ranen NG, Nance MA, Paulsen JS. A physician's guide to the management of Huntington's disease, 2nd edition. Huntington's Disease Society of America, New York, 1999.

University of Montana Practical Ethics Centre: *Lifting the Veil of Huntington's Disease*. Huntington's Disease Workgroup Recommendations to the Field. [Available on-line from www.promotingexcellence.org]

Cerebral tumour

Krouwer HGT, Pallagi JL, Graves NM. Management of seizures in brain tumor patients at the end of life. *Journal of Palliative Medicine* 2000; 3(4): 465–7.

Ethical issues

Advance directives

Thompson TD, Barbour RS, Schwartz L. Health professionals' views on advance directives: a qualitative interdisciplinary study. *Palliative Medicine* 2003; 17(5): 403–9.

Minimal conscious state (MCS)

Giacino JT, Ashwal S, Childs N, Cranford R, Jennet B, Katz DI, Kelly JP, Rosenberg JH, Whyte J, Zafonte RD, Zasler ND. The minimally conscious state. Definition and diagnostic criteria. *Neurology* 2002; 58: 349–53.

Persistent vegetative state (PVS)

Practice Parameters: Assessment and Management of Patients in the Persistent Vegetative State (Summary Statement). Report of the Quality Standards Subcommittee of the American Academy of Neurology. *Neurology* 1995; 45: 1015–18.

Sazbon L, Zagreba F, Ronen J, Solzi P, Costeff H. Course and outcome of patients in vegetative state of nontraumatic aetiology. *Journal of Neurology Neurosurgery and Psychiatry* 1993; 56(4): 407–9.

Young B, Blume W, Lynch A. Brain death and the persistent vegetative state: similarities and contrasts. *Canadian Journal of Neurological Sciences* 1989; 16: 388–93.

Terminal sedation

Dresser R. The Supreme Court and end-of-life care: principled distinctions or slippery slope? In: Schneider CE. *Law at the End of Life: The Supreme Court and Assisted Suicide*. Cambridge University Press, Cambridge, 2000.
[Discusses ethical and legal distinctions between terminal sedation and assisted suicide.]

Criteria for an effective Palliation Service

Lynn J, Schuster JL, Kabcenell A. *Improving Care for the End of Life: A Sourcebook for Health Care Managers and Clinicians*. Cambridge University Press, Cambridge, 2000.

Mathew A, Cowley S, Bliss J, Thistlewood G. The development of palliative care in national government policy in England, 1986–2000. *Palliative Medicine* 2003; 17(3): 270–82.

4

Medications

Medications referred to in this text are as follows.

Drug	Formulation	Dose range	Common use
A			
Acetylcysteine	20% solution	2 ml in nebulizer	For inhalation as mucolytic; retained secretions
Alprazolam	0.25 mg tab.	0.25–0.5 mg tab.	Anxiolytic
Alprostadil	10, 20 mg amp.	10–20 mg	Intracavernosal injection for erectile failure
Amantadine	100 mg tab.	Once or twice daily	Fatigue in MS
Amisulpride	50, 100 mg tab.	50–800 mg/day	Antipsychotic, less Parkinsonism, Huntington's
Amitriptyline	10, 25, 75 mg tab.; 25, 75 mg/5 ml susp.	10–200 mg at night	Antidepressant, neuropathic pain
Amphotericin	Lozenges 10 mg	One qid	Oral candidiasis
Apomorphine	50 mg amp.	Up to 50 mg/24 h	Dopamine receptor agonist; Parkinson's disease
Atropine	0.6 mg amp.	qid; 1.2 mg/24-h infusion	Anticholinergic, dry-up oral secretions
Azathioprine	150 mg tab.	1 daily	Antimetabolite, treatment of CIDP
Azithromycin	500 mg tab.	500 mg daily	Treatment of *M. avium* infection in HIV disease
B			
Baclofen	5 mg tab., 0.05 mg/ml pack	5–30 mg bd–qid	Oral antispasmodic; intrathecal dose 100–300 µg
Benzhexol	2, 5 mg tab.	Up to 10 mg daily	Treatment of acute dystonic reactions
Benztropine	2 mg tab., amp.	0.5–2 mg/24 h, oral, I-M or I-V	Treatment of acute dystonic reactions
Bifanazole	Cream	Apply daily, bd	Antifungal topical cream
Biperiden	2 mg tab.	1–4 mg/day	Treatment of acute dystonic reactions
Bisacodyl	5 mg tab.	2–4 daily up to tds	Aperient
Bromocriptine	2.5 mg tab., 5 mg cap.	2.5–15 mg bd	Dopamine agonist, Parkinson's disease
Botulinum toxin	Injection	20–50 U	Blocks acetylcholine, treatment of muscle spasm
Bupivicaine	0.25–0.5% solution	1–5 ml up to tds	Local anaesthetic, spinal route in severe pain

C

Drug	Formulation	Dose	Indication
Cabergoline	0.5 mg tab.	Up to 5 mg once daily	Dopamine agonist, Parkinson's disease
Cannabis [tetrahydrocannabinol]	2.5 mg tab.	2.5–15 mg/day	Dry leaf smoked, cooked in biscuits enhance appetite, treat nausea
Capsaicin	0.075% cream	Four times daily topical	Neuralgic pain and allodynia
Carbamazepine	100, 200 mg tab.; 200, 400 mg CR	To 1000 mg daily	Neuropathic pain
Carbidopa–levodopa	25, 50 mg carbidopa; 100–250 mg levodopa	Dose variable	Parkinson's disease
Chlorpromazine	25, 100 mg tab.; 25 mg/5 ml susp.; 50 mg/2 ml amp.	50–300 mg in 24 h	Hiccups, sedation
Cholestyramine	4–6 g powder	12–16 g/day	Exchange resin, cholestasis pruritus
Cimetidine	200, 400, 800 mg tab.; 200 mg amp.	Up to 1200 mg/day	Histamine H_2-receptor antagonist, gastro-oesophageal reflux, smaller dose reduces sweating
Cisapride	5 mg tab.	5–10 mg before meals	Anti-emetic, assists gastric emptying
Citalopram	20 mg tab.	20–60 mg at night	SSRI antidepressant; pseudobulbar disease in ALS
Clonazepam	0.5, 2 mg tab.; 1 mg amp.	2–6 mg/day	Anti-epileptic, anxiolytic
Clonidine	100, 150 µg tab.; 150 µg amp.	50–100 µg oral, S/C, intraspinal	Antihypertensive, neuropathic pain
Clotrimazole	1% cream	Topical bd–tds	Candidiasis and dermatophytosis
Clozapine	25, 100 mg tab.	12.5–400 mg/day	Antipsychotic
Codeine	30 mg tab.	1–2 tab., 4 hourly	Analgesic
Cotrimoxazole	Trimethoprim 160 mg, sulphamethoxazole 800 mg	1 tab. bd	Anti-infective, HIV
Cyclizine	50 mg amp.	100–150-mg/day infusion	Nausea, gastric stasis
Cyproheptadine	4 mg tab.	To 12 mg/day	Antihistamine, appetite support in anorexia

(continued)

Drug	Formulation	Dose range	Common use
D			
Dantrolene	25 mg tab.	Up to 400 mg/day	Spasticity, especially of central origin
Desmopressin	Nasal spray 10 μg	One each nostril daily	Antidiuretic hormone, reduce nocturia
Dextromethorphan	10–15 mg/5 ml susp.	10–15 mg tds	Cough suppressant
Diamorphine	5, 10, 30, 100, 500 mg inj.	No fixed, upper dose	Major opioid, used mainly in UK
			Commonly used in syringe-drivers
Diazepam	2, 5, 10 mg tab.	5–10 mg oral	Anxiolytic
	10 mg amp.	10–20 mg I-V	To abort acute seizure
Dicyclomine	10 mg tab.	10–20 mg tds	Antispasmodic, reduces bladder contraction
Dimenhydrinate	1 mg/ml susp.	50–400 mg/day	Sedating antihistamine, anti-emetic
	50 mg tab.	2–8/day	Constipation
Docusate 50 mg + senna 8 mg	Tab.		
Docusate	120 mg tab.	2–8/day	Constipation
Domperidone	10 mg tab.	10–20 mg tds	Anti-emetic, less risk of dyskinesic reaction
Donepezil	5 mg tab.	5–10 mg/day	Anticholinesterase inhibitor, dementia
Doxepin	25 mg tab.	25–150 mg/day	Tricyclic antidepressant, H$_1$-histamine receptor antagonist
Doxepin	5% cream	Topical prn	For management of itch
Droperidol	2.5, 10 mg amp.	2.5–10 mg up to tds	Agitation, delirium
E			
Enoxaparin	20, 40, 60, 80, 100 U	30–100 U/daily dose	Prevention, treatment, pulmonary embolus
Esomeprazole	40 mg tab.	1 daily	Histamine H$_2$-receptor antagonist
Ethambutol	100, 400 mg tab.	25 mg/kg daily 2 months, then 15 mg/kg daily	Anti-infective; *M. avium* complex, HIV

F		
Famotidine	20 mg tab.	1 twice daily	Histamine H_2-receptor antagonist; gastro-oesophageal reflux
Fentanyl	Transdermal patch, 2.5–10.0 mg	Re-apply each 2–3 days	Transdermal opioid; baseline analgesia
Fentanyl lozenge	200–1600 µg	Apply to gum prn	For break-through pain
Flecainide	100 mg tab., 10 mg/ml	50–200 mg bd	Antidysrhythmia; used in neuropathic pain
Fluconazole	100, 150, 200 mg tab.	50–400 mg daily	Candidiasis
	100-mg infusion	200–400 mg daily	Cryptococcal meningitis
Flumazenil	0.5 mg amp.	0.2 mg up to 1 mg I-V	For reversal of acute benzodiazepine sedation
Fluoxetine	20 mg tab.	20–60 mg/day	SSRI antidepressant
Frusemide	20, 40 mg tab., amp.	20–400 mg daily	Diuretic
G		
Gabapentin	300, 400 mg tab.	600–2400 mg/day	Epilepsy, neuropathic pain
Galantamine	4 mg tab.	4–8 mg bd	Cholinesterase inhibitor, dementia
Ganciclovir	250, 500 mg tab.	5 mg/kg I-V, 12 hourly	Anti-infective
	500-mg infusion	For 2–3 weeks	Cytomegalovirus retinitis, AIDS
Glatiramer acetate	20 mg S/C inj.	Daily	Immune modulation, MS
Glycopyrrolate	0.2 mg amp.		
	0.2–0.4 mg S/C, 4 hourly	1.2 mg/24-h infusion	Suppress excess oral secretions
H		
Haloperidol	0.5, 1.5, 5 mg tab. 5 mg amp.	0.5–10 mg–30 mg/day	Antipsychotic, anti-emetic
Hydromorphone	Susp., 1 mg/ml 2, 4, 8 mg tab. 2 mg, 10 mg/ml amp.	No dose range	Major opioid Also CR tab. in some countries
Hyoscine hydrobromide	0.4 mg amp.	0.4–0.6 mg, 4–6 hourly	Suppress excess oral secretions

(continued)

Drug	Formulation	Dose range	Common use
I			
Ibuprofen	200, 400 mg tab.	200–400 mg bd–tds	NSAID chronic inflammation pain
Imipramine	25 mg tab.	25–50 mg at night	Antidepressant, promote sleep
Interferon beta	6 milliunits or 22 μg	Three times weekly	Immune modulator, MS
Ipatropium	250 μg/ml solution	Nebulizer prn qid	To assist clearing bronchial secretions
K			
Ketamine	1–10 mg/ml solution	20–50 mg bolus S/C	NMDA receptor antagonist
		100–600-mg/24-h infusion	Neuropathic and difficult pain
Ketoconazole	200 mg tab.	200 mg daily	Oral candidiasis resisting topical therapy
L			
Lactulose	Solution	10–30 ml, 2–3 times/day	Osmotic aperient; constipation
Lamotrigine	25, 50, 100, 200 tab.	50–200 mg bd	Anticonvulsant; neuropathic pain
Lansoprazole	30 mg tab.	1 daily	Proton pump inhibitor; gastro-oesophageal reflux
Lignocaine	1%, 2% solution	1–2 g/24-h S/C infusion	Local anaesthetic; neuropathic pain
Lithium carbonate	250 mg tab.; 450 mg slow release	0.25–1 g daily	Mood stabilizer, pseudobulbar disease in ALS
Loperamide	2 mg tab.	Up to 16 mg/day	Antidiarrhoeal
Lorazepam	2 mg tab.	2–4 mg to sleep	Anxiolytic

M

Drug	Formulation	Dose	Notes
Macrogol	13 g sachet	1–4 sachets daily	Constipation
Magnesium oxide	Powder	One teaspoon in water bd–tds	Constipation
Medroxyprogesterone acetate	100–500 mg tab.	1 daily	Appetite encouragement
Megestrol acetate	40 mg tab.	40–160 mg daily	Appetite encouragement
Methadone	5 mg/ml solution, 10 mg tab., 10 mg/ml amp.	No dose range*	Major opioid, variable long half-life
Methylphenidate	10 mg tab.	10 mg a.m. and midday	Psychostimulant, drowsiness, fatigue
Methylprednisolone	500 mg, 1 g pack	1 g/day	Corticosteroid; acute relapse of MS
Metoclopramide	10 mg tab., amp.	10–20 mg up to qid	Antinausea, anti-emetic
Mexiletine	50, 200 mg cap.	50–200 mg tds	Antidysrhythmia, neuropathic pain
Morphine	Susp.: 1, 2, 5, 10 mg/ml; CR tab.: 5, 10, 20, 30, 50, 60, 100, 200 mg; Injection: 5, 10, 15, 30 mg (sulphate), 120 mg (tartrate)	Oral dose approximately three times injected dose; up to 20 times intrathecal dose	Major opioid
Miconazole	2% cream, gel, powder	Topical bd–qid	Antifungal, anticandida
Midazolam	5, 15 mg amp.	2.5–120 mg daily	Sedative, anxiolytic, useful as bolus and continuous infusion
Mirtazepine	30, 45 mg tab.	30–60 mg/day	Antidepressant
Misoprostol	200 µg tab.	2–4/day	Prostaglandin E analogue; protects gastric mucosa
Modafinil	100 mg tab.	400 mg daily	Improve fatigue in MS

(continued)

Drug	Formulation	Dose range	Common use
N			
Naloxone	0.4, 0.8, 2 mg pre-filled syringe	Slow injection S/C, I-V	Opioid antagonist
Naproxen	250, 500 mg tab.; 750, 1 g CR tab.	To 1.5 g daily	NSAID inflammatory pain
Nifedipine	10 mg tab.	10–20 mg tds	Ca channel blocker, muscle relaxant: hiccups
Nortriptyline	10, 25 mg tab.	10–150 mg/day	Non-sedating antidepressant
Nystatin	100 000 U/ml	1 ml orally, qid	Oral candidiasis
O			
Octreotide	50, 100 μg amp.	50–300 μg bd	Somatostatin analogue; diarrhoea in AIDS
Olanzapine	2.5, 5, 7.5, 10 mg tab.; 5, 10 mg oral wafers	5–20 mg/day	Antipsychotic
Omeprazole	10, 20 mg tab.	10–40 mg/day	Proton pump inhibitor; gastric ulcer, gastro-oesophageal reflux
Ondansetron	4, 8 mg tab., amp.	4–16 mg/day	Nausea and vomiting after chemotherapy
Orphenadrine	100 mg tab.	100 mg bd or tds	Antispasmodic; muscle spasms
Oxazepam	15, 30 mg tab.	15–30 mg, 1–3/day	Sedative, anxiolytic
Oxybutynin	5 mg tab.	2.5–5 mg tds	Antispasmodic, urinary urgency
Oxycodone			
Immediate release tab.:	5, 10, 20 mg	No set dose range	Major opioid; ampoules for injection available in some countries
Sustained-release tab.:	10, 20, 40, 80 mg		

P

Drug	Formulation	Dose	Indication
Pantoprazole	20, 40 mg tab., 40 mg amp.	20–40 mg daily, bd	Proton pump inhibitor; gastric ulcer, gastro-oesophageal reflux
Pentothal sodium	0.5 g amp.	0.5–1.5 g slow I-V	Anaesthetic induction
Pergolide	50, 100 μg, 1 mg tab.	50 μg–1 mg bd	Adjunct to L-dopa therapy, Parkinson's disease
Pericyazine	2.5, 10 mg tab.	5–30 mg/day	Severe anxiety, psychosis
Phenobarbitone	300 mg amp.	200–600 mg S/C bolus	Sedation, epilepsy
Phenytoin sodium	30, 100 mg tab.; 100, 250 mg amp.	300–600 mg daily	Epilepsy, neuropathic pain
Pholcodine	1 mg/ml susp.	15 mg qid prn	Cough suppressant
Prochlorperazine	5 mg tab., 12.5 mg amp.; 5, 25 mg suppository	5–10 mg tds	Antinausea, anti-emetic, vertigo
Propantheline	15 mg tab.	7.5–30 mg tds	Anticholinergic, urinary incontinence
propranolol	10, 40, 160 mg tab.	10–240 mg daily	Beta-blocker, essential tremor
Prazosin	1, 2, 5 mg tab.	2 mg bd	Benign prostatic hypertrophy
Primidone	250 mg tab.	125–750 mg twice daily	Anticonvulsant
Promethazine theoclate	25 mg tab.	Up to 100 mg in 24 h	Antinausea, anti-emetic
Propofol	200, 500, 1 g vial	Up to 10 mg/h	Strong sedation for severe agitation

Q

Drug	Formulation	Dose	Indication
Quinine	300 mg tab.	300 mg at night	Prevention of night cramps

R

Drug	Formulation	Dose	Indication
Ranitidine	150, 300 mg tab.	150–300 mg daily, tds	H_2-receptor antagonist, peptic ulcer
Rabeprazole	10, 20 mg tab.	10–20 mg daily, bd	Proton pump inhibitor, gastro-oesophageal reflux

(continued)

Drug	Formulation	Dose range	Common use
Rifampicin	150, 300 mg tab.; 600 mg vial	450–600 mg/day	Mycobacterial infection
Rifabutin	150 mg tab.	Complex	Mycobacterial infection in HIV
Riluzole	50 mg tab.	50–100 mg daily	Glutamate antagonist ALS (MND)
Rivastigmine	1.5, 3, 4.5, 6 mg cap.	1.5–6 mg bd	Initial treatment Alzheimer's disease
Risperidone	1, 2, 3, 4 mg tab.	0.25–1 mg bd	Dementia restlessness, aggression
	1 mg/ml vial	2–6 mg/day	Acute psychosis
	25–50 mg ER vial	25–50 mg every 2 weeks	Pychosis maintenance
S			
Salbutamol	5 mg/ml vial	2.5–5 mg by nebulizer	Bronchodilator, assist clearing of bronchial secretions
	2.5, 5 mg nebule	up to qid	
Sertraline	50, 100 mg tab.	50–200 mg daily	SSRI antidepressant
Sildenafil	25, 50, 100 mg tab.	25–100 mg, 1 h before sex	Erectile dysfunction in male
Simvastatin	10, 20, 40, 80 mg tab.	80 mg daily	To improve deterioration in MS
Sorbitol	70% liquid	10–30 ml daily, tds	Osmotic agent for constipation
Sulpride (see amisulpride)			
Suxamethonium chloride	100 mg/2 ml amp.	0.3–1 mg/kg I-V	Muscle relaxant in anaesthesia
T			
Tadalafil	10, 20 mg tab.	10–20 mg prior to sex	Erectile dysfunction
Temazepam	10, 20 mg tab.	10–30 mg at night	Night sedation

Tetrabenazine	25 mg tab.	25–100 mg bd	Huntington's disease
Tetrahydrocannabinol tablets		2.5–15 mg/day	Antinausea, improve appetite
Terazosin	1, 2, 5, 10 mg tab.	1–10 mg daily	Benign prostatic hypertrophy
Thioridazine	10 mg tab.	1 at night	Prevent night sweats
	50, 100 mg tab., susp.	50–100 mg, 2 hourly to 300 mg	Psychosis
Tizanidine	4 mg tab.	4–18 mg/day	Reducing muscle spasm
Topiramate	25, 50, 100, 200 mg tab., 200 mg/5 ml susp.	25–500 mg/day	Anticonvulsant

V

| Valproate sodium | 100, 200, 500 mg tab. | 400 mg–2 g/day | Prevention of seizures; neuropathic pain |
| Venlafaxine | 37.5, 75 mg tab., 75, 150 mg cap. | 75–375 mg/day | Antidepressant |

Z

Zolpidem	10 mg tab.	10 mg at night	Short-term treatment of insomnia
Zopiclone	7.5 mg tab.	3.75–7.5 mg at night	Short-term treatment of insomnia
Zuclopenthixol acetate	10, 25 mg tab.	10–50 mg/day	Antipsychotic
	50 mg amp.	50–400 mg I-M/day	Acute psychosis
	200mg amp.	100–200mg/2–4 weeks	Maintenance treatment

AIDS: acquired immune deficiency syndrome; ALS: amyotrophic lateral sclerosis; CIDP: chronic inflammatory demyelinating polyneuropathy; HIV: human immunodeficiency virus; MND: motor neurone disease; MS: multiple sclerosis; NMDA: N-methyl-D-aspartate; NSAID: non-steroidal anti-inflammatory drug; SSRI: selective serotonin reuptake inhibitors; I-M: intramuscular; I-V: intravenous; M. avium: Mycobacterium avium.

Index